# THE COMPLETE BOOK OF
# PALEO COOKING

Publications International, Ltd.

**Pictured on the front cover:** Beef and Beet Borscht *(page 272)*.

**Pictured on the back cover** *(clockwise from left):* Chicken Scarpiello *(page 64)*, Mustard-Grilled Red Snapper *(page 159)* and Marinated Beef Brochettes *(page 86)*.

ISBN: 978-1-64030-450-5

Manufactured in China.

8 7 6 5 4 3 2 1

**Microwave Cooking:** Microwave ovens vary in wattage. Use the cooking times as guidelines and check for doneness before adding more time.

# CONTENTS

# A NEW DIET THAT'S 100,000 YEARS OLD:
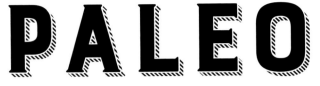

Humans were hunter-gatherers for tens of thousands of years. They ate the wild plants they could find and the meat they could kill. Why should we care what they ate? One reason is that after all these centuries, our DNA is still virtually identical to theirs.

The most profound and recent change in the way humans live and eat resulted from the invention of agriculture, which began less than 10,000 years ago—a mere drop in the bucket in evolutionary history. Agriculture allowed us to go from a diet of lean meat and lots of different kinds of fruits and vegetables to one based primarily on grains and starchy crops.

There is quite a lot of anthropological evidence that this change was not healthy for Homo sapiens. Studies of early agricultural societies indicate that they had shorter life spans, more malnutrition and were shorter in stature than their Paleolithic forebears. Agriculture allowed us to stay in one place, to feed more people and to develop culture. Nobody wants to go back to the Stone Age. But since our genetic make-up hasn't changed, maybe, just maybe, the modern high-carb, low-fat diet isn't the ideal for us.

## PALEO MADE SIMPLE

1. Eat whole foods, not processed

2. Don't eat grains (especially wheat, but also corn, rice, oats, barley)

3. Eliminate dairy products

4. Avoid legumes (beans, peanuts)

5. Enjoy lots of vegetables and plenty of protein

## BUT I'M NOT A CAVEMAN!

Our lives are (thank heavens!) very different, but our digestive systems may not be. Obviously we can't literally eat what Paleo man did. Nobody wants to dine on bison brain with a side of bitter greens. What the Paleo diet proposes is that we learn from what worked and find modern healthy equivalents. It's not complicated. It's an invitation to change your diet from mostly processed, refined carbohydrates to whole foods, protein, carbohydrates from fruits and vegetables, and good fats.

# THE PALEO PANTRY

## WHAT'S IN:

**MEATS:** Bacon, Beef, Buffalo, Lamb, Pork, Veal, Venison

**POULTRY:** Chicken, Duck, Quail, Turkey

**EGGS** (preferably organic and pasture-raised)

**SEAFOOD:** Catfish, Clams, Halibut, Herring, Lobster, Mahimahi, Mussels, Salmon, Sardines, Scallops, Shrimp, Trout, Tuna

**FATS AND OILS:** Butter (grass-fed), Coconut oil, Nut oils, Olive oil, Palm oil

**VEGETABLES:** Artichokes, Arugula, Asparagus, Broccoli, Brussels sprouts, Cabbage, Carrots, Cauliflower, Celery, Chard, Cucumbers, Eggplant, Fennel, Garlic, Green beans, Kale, Kohlrabi, Leeks, Lettuce, Mushrooms, Onions, Parsnips, Peppers, Radishes, Rutabagas, Spinach, Squash, Sweet potatoes, Tomatoes

**FRUITS:** Apricots, Avocados, Bananas, Blackberries, Blueberries, Cherries, Coconut, Cranberries, Figs, Grapefruit, Grapes, Kiwis, Lemons, Limes, Mangoes, Melons, Nectarines, Oranges, Papayas, Peaches, Pears, Pineapples, Plums, Pomegranates, Raspberries, Rhubarb, Strawberries, Tangerines, Watermelon

**NUTS AND SEEDS:** Almonds, Brazil nuts, Hazelnuts, Macadamia nuts, Pecans, Pine nuts, Pistachios, Pumpkin seeds, Sesame seeds, Sunflower seeds, Walnuts

**FLAVORINGS:** Capers, Coconut aminos, Fresh and dried herbs, Ginger, Lemon and lime juice, Mustard, Vanilla, Vinegars (balsamic, cider, wine), Whole and ground spices

## WHAT'S OUT:

**PROCESSED FOODS**

**GRAINS:** Barley, Corn, Oats, Millet, Quinoa, Rice, Rye, Wheat and products containing them or containing gluten

**PREPARED/PACKAGED CARBS:** Bagels, Baked goods, Biscuits, Breads, Breakfast and snack bars, Cereal, Chips, Cookies, Crackers, Muffins, Pasta, Pretzels, Scones, Tacos

**DAIRY:** Cheese, Ice cream, Milk, Yogurt (see page 9 for exceptions)

**LEGUMES:** Beans, Chickpeas, Soybeans and soy products, Peanuts

**PROCESSED VEGETABLE OILS:** Canola oil, Corn oil, Margarine and "buttery" spreads, Peanut oil, Shortening, Vegetable oil

**SUGAR AND ARTIFICIAL SWEETENERS:** Brown, cane and powdered sugar, Corn syrup, Dextrose, Sucrose or products containing them

# SO WHAT'S FOR DINNER
## (AND BREAKFAST AND LUNCH)?

A glance at the Paleo pantry and the many wonderful recipes in this book should give you some good ideas. If you've been eating a typical modern diet of fast food, pasta, bread and sweets, Paleo does take adjustments. You'll spend more time shopping and cooking and being mindful of what you eat—and that's a good thing.

## EAT ENOUGH PROTEIN

Meat (especially red meat), poultry and eggs have been maligned for years since they contain cholesterol and saturated fat. They do, but as you have probably noticed, nutritional guidelines change over time. Once egg yolks were forbidden because they raised cholesterol. Then we learned that there are many kinds of cholesterol that your body needs and what we eat may not increase the amount in our bloodstreams. Will eating red meat put you in immediate danger of a heart attack? Not so fast. It depends on what else you're eating, what kind of meat it is and dozens of other factors.

### WHAT'S THE DIFFERENCE BETWEEN PALEO, LOW CARB AND GLUTEN-FREE?

There are similarities, but the basic premise of the Paleo diet is to eat only whole, unprocessed foods. Most low-carb regimens are designed for quick weight loss and require limiting some fruits and vegetables. Gluten-free diets are for those with celiac disease or other sensitivities to the protein in wheat.

To stick to the Paleo plan you need the simplest, highest quality protein you can find and afford. The best choices are pasture-raised, grass-fed meat and eggs. This is easy to understand if you remember that animals raised on a feedlot and fattened on corn are not remotely like the lean, free-range animals our ancestors consumed.

Pasture-raised meat contains a larger proportion of beneficial omega-3 fatty acids, the same helpful nutrient that is in fish oil and is sadly lacking in the modern diet. When choosing supermarket meat, go for leaner cuts. Most importantly, avoid any processed product that has been "enhanced," marinated or pre-seasoned. Look for eggs from chickens that are fed a diet that increases the content of omega-3s where pasture-raised is hard to find or too expensive.

When choosing seafood, the closer it is to its natural state, the better. If you can't go fishing yourself, look for wild-caught fish and purchase from a reputable source that has a high turnover. Pay attention to country of origin when purchasing shrimp. The best choice is U.S. farmed. Imported products can be raised in polluted waters.

## ENJOY LOTS OF VEGETABLES AT BREAKFAST, LUNCH AND DINNER

No need to count calories or carbs when it comes to vegetables. It's practically impossible to overeat broccoli or salad greens. Most Paleo diets eliminate potatoes, but sweet potatoes are permitted. (They're botanically unrelated to white potatoes.)

Take this opportunity to try new and different vegetables. How about a frittata with fresh spinach for breakfast? Dress up your lunchtime salad with artichoke hearts. Make crunchy chips from beets or kale for a snack. Roast parsnips, carrots and rutabaga drizzled with olive oil as a side dish. Add fennel, sweet peppers and onions to roast chicken.

Choose local, seasonal and organic produce whenever possible. Some vegetables and fruits are more likely to be contaminated with pesticide residue than others; choosing organic can limit your exposure in those cases. Some of the items more likely to be contaminated include strawberries, spinach, nectarines, apples, grapes, peaches, cherries, pears, tomatoes, celery and bell peppers.

## CHOOSE THE RIGHT KINDS OF FATS

By now you've probably accepted that it's not fat that makes us fat. Our fat storage system is dependent on insulin, and insulin levels increase in response to carbohydrates. Still, the kind of fat we eat does matter. The saturated fat found in red meat used to be considered unhealthy, but that's certainly what Paleo man ate. There were no manufactured vegetable oils.

Did we improve on nature by switching from saturated fat to polyunsaturated vegetable oils? Probably not. What we did do was drastically change the ratio of omega-3 fatty acids to omega-6 fatty acids in our diets. Omega-3s come from grass-fed meats and wild-caught fish. Vegetable oils, including corn, canola and soy, are the primary source of excess omega-6 fatty acids today. This lack of balance is the reason for the increasing interest in fish oil capsules and flaxseed, which are high in omega-3s.

What this means is that you should avoid processed polyunsaturated oils and, of course, trans fats. Instead use olive oil, coconut oil, avocado oil, macadamia nut oil or butter from pasture-raised cows. Wherever possible, eat grass-fed meats instead of corn-fed factory-farmed animals.

### COCONUT AMINOS

Made from the sap of the coconut palm, this bottled product is an excellent replacement for soy sauce. In addition to being made from soy beans, traditional soy sauce also has added wheat, so it contains gluten. Coconut aminos can be used in stir-fries, dressings and wherever you would use soy sauce.

## KEEP THINGS INTERESTING WITH NUTS, SEEDS, HERBS AND SPICES

Making meals and snacks pleasurable doesn't have to mean spending more money or time. Almond or macadamia butter can easily replace peanut butter with your sliced apples. Herbs and spices can add endless variation to the simplest preparations. Herbs and spices are all paleo, but watch ingredient lists if you're purchasing prepared blends. They often contain sugar in some form.

## GIVING UP GRAIN

How can wheat, corn, soy, oats, rice and rye be bad for us? They are all domesticated forms of wild grasses that have been managed and "improved" by agriculture for 5,000 years. Remember, that's a short time in terms of human evolution. Wheat, barley and rye contain a protein called gluten. Other grains have similar but somewhat less problematic proteins.

Long ago humans lived without grain. Today our diets are dominated by it. We eat a muffin for breakfast, a sandwich for lunch and a bowl of pasta for dinner. There's a lot of hidden gluten, soy and corn in processed foods as well. It's used to improve the texture of everything from hot dogs to ketchup. Corn appears as high fructose corn syrup among other manufactured additives. Soy lurks in snack foods, cooking oils and most dairy replacement products. Start reading labels and you will be stunned at the amount of grain you consume without being aware of it.

### HOW ABOUT WHOLE GRAINS?

Sorry! While whole grains have a better nutritional profile than refined grains, they contain the same anti-nutrients and can cause the same problems.

## GRAINS ARE EASY TO SWALLOW, BUT HARD TO DIGEST

Grain is hard on our digestive system because it contains anti-nutrients. From a plant's perspective these are defensive mechanisms. Plants can't run away from a predator so they evolved chemical protections to make them less attractive as food and to keep them viable. What protects a plant's seeds also protects it from easy digestion, so for humans that makes it an anti-nutrient. One of the many (and most studied) of grains' anti-nutrients is lectin. It occurs in virtually all plants to varying degrees, but is much more concentrated in grain. Lectins are not broken down enough to easily pass into your bloodstream as smaller molecules, so they can compromise the lining of your intestines and cause everything from food intolerances to autoimmune diseases.

## WHERE WILL I GET CALCIUM WITHOUT DAIRY?

There are plenty of foods, including dark green leafy vegetables, that supply calcium. More importantly, the body's ability to absorb calcium depends on other nutrients, especially magnesium and vitamin K2, which can come from a variety of vegetable sources. Phytate, an anti-nutrient present in wheat, can also bind with calcium and prevent absorption.

## BUT WE NEED CARBS!

Sure we do, but we don't need all the starch and sugar we consume today. We eat a lot more bad carbs than our grandparents did. Carbohydrates are broken down into glucose (sugar) quickly in the bloodstream. If you eat more than you need, your body stores the excess as fat.

There are many sources of good carbs that aren't grain. Fruits and nuts are high in carbohydrates. So are many vegetables including sweet potatoes, carrots and winter squash. They also contribute a wide range of nutrients to your diet.

## SAY BYE-BYE TO BEANS

Digesting beans presents most of the same problems as grain. Beans, peanuts (not a nut, but a legume), soybeans and lentils have anti-nutrients just like grains. Like grains, they are difficult to digest. That's why they cause gas. Soaking, fermenting and cooking beans reduces the level of lectins but doesn't remove them. In fact, red kidney beans have such a high concentration of lectin that if they are not thoroughly cooked, they can cause illness. Several outbreaks have been associated with beans prepared in a slow cooker when the temperature was not high enough.

## DON'T DO (MOST) DAIRY

Hunter-gatherers certainly didn't have a herd of milk cows following them around. Most of the dairy products we use are highly processed and come from grain-fed cows. They're ultra-pasteurized, homogenized and then fortified to replace nutrients that have been lost. Skim and reduced-fat milk have more lactose, which is milk sugar, because that's what's left when the fat is removed. Lactose intolerance is common. Butter or cream from pasture-raised animals is usually well tolerated since it contains fewer irritating proteins and almost no lactose.

## BUT WE NEED FIBER!

Paleo man consumed a great deal of fiber from wild greens and fruits, not from grains or legumes. Following the Paleo path means eating a lot more fruits and vegetables than our modern, grain-heavy diet provides. You'll be getting fiber from avocados, broccoli, carrots and greens instead of a sweet bran muffin or a processed breakfast cereal.

## GET SAUCY

Eating Paleo doesn't have to be boring or restrictive—there's more to meals than just meat and vegetables! But you might need to find new ways to add flavor to your food because so many supermarket sauces and condiments are loaded with sugar, corn syrup and other processed ingredients. Read labels carefully—or better yet, make your own. Many basic Paleo sauces can be made in minutes; store them in the refrigerator so you can use them for your everyday cooking (including recipes in this book).

### PALEO WORCESTERSHIRE SAUCE
Makes about ¾ cup

½ cup cider vinegar
2 tablespoons water
2 tablespoons coconut aminos
1 teaspoon fish sauce
1 teaspoon molasses
¼ teaspoon onion powder
¼ teaspoon garlic powder
¼ teaspoon ground mustard
⅛ teaspoon ground cinnamon
⅛ teaspoon black pepper
Pinch ground cloves

Combine all ingredients in small saucepan; bring to a boil over medium heat. Reduce heat to low; simmer 3 minutes. Cool to room temperature; refrigerate up to 1 month.

### TANGY BARBECUE SAUCE
Makes about 2 cups

1 can (15 ounces) tomato sauce
⅔ cup water
½ cup cider vinegar
3 tablespoons honey
2 tablespoons maple syrup
1 teaspoon salt
1 teaspoon onion powder
1 teaspoon smoked paprika
½ teaspoon garlic powder
½ teaspoon black pepper

Combine all ingredients in small saucepan; bring to a simmer over medium heat. Reduce heat to low; simmer 30 to 40 minutes or until slightly thickened, stirring occasionally. Cool to room temperature; refrigerate up to 2 weeks.

## PALEO HOISIN SAUCE
### Makes ¾ cup

½ cup coconut aminos
¼ cup sunflower seed butter
   or almond butter
2 tablespoons molasses
2 teaspoons cider vinegar

2 teaspoons tomato paste
1 teaspoon sesame oil
1 teaspoon garlic powder
½ teaspoon Chinese five-spice
   powder

Whisk all ingredients in medium bowl until smooth. Refrigerate up to
2 weeks.

---

## CLASSIC SALSA
### Makes about 2 cups

3 medium plum tomatoes,
   seeded and chopped
2 tablespoons chopped onion
1 small jalapeño pepper,*
   seeded and minced
1 tablespoon chopped
   fresh cilantro

1 tablespoon lime juice
¼ teaspoon salt
⅛ teaspoon black pepper

*Jalapeño peppers can sting and
irritate the skin, so wear rubber
gloves when handling peppers
and do not touch your eyes.*

Combine tomatoes, onion, jalapeño, cilantro, lime juice, salt and black
pepper in small bowl. Refrigerate until ready to serve.

---

## AVOCADO SALSA
### Makes about 4 cups

1 medium avocado, diced
1 cup chopped onion
1 cup peeled seeded
   chopped cucumber
1 Anaheim pepper, seeded
   and chopped
½ cup chopped fresh tomato

2 tablespoons chopped fresh
   cilantro, plus additional
   for garnish
½ teaspoon salt
¼ teaspoon hot pepper sauce

Combine all ingredients in medium bowl; mix gently. Cover and refrigerate
at least 1 hour before serving. Garnish with additional cilantro.

## DRESS IT UP

If you crave ranch dressing for your salad or a little ketchup for your meat loaf, don't despair. The bottles you find on supermarket shelves might not be Paleo approved, but the homemade versions are quick and easy.

## PALEO MAYONNAISE
### Makes about 1½ cups

1¼ cups light olive oil or avocado oil, divided (do not use extra virgin olive oil)

1 egg,* at room temperature

½ teaspoon salt

½ teaspoon mustard powder

1 tablespoon lemon juice

*Use very fresh organic eggs or pasteurized eggs, as the egg is not cooked in this recipe.

**1.** Combine ¼ cup oil, egg, salt and mustard powder in food processor or blender; process until well blended.

**2.** With motor running, very slowly and steadily drizzle in remaining 1 cup oil through feed tube. (Oil must be added gradually; entire process should take 1 to 2 minutes.) Stir in lemon juice until blended. Store covered in refrigerator up to 1 month.

**TIPS:** It's important that the ingredients be at room temperature to emulsify the eggs and oil. The oil should be added as slowly as possible—the slower it is added, the thicker the mayonnaise will be. You can also use an immersion blender instead.

## PALEO RANCH DRESSING
### Makes about 1¼ cups

1 cup Paleo Mayonnaise (see recipe above)

1 tablespoon chopped fresh parsley

1 tablespoon chopped fresh chives

1 teaspoon lemon juice

½ teaspoon dried dill weed

¼ teaspoon onion powder

¼ teaspoon salt

⅛ teaspoon ground black pepper

1 to 2 tablespoons coconut milk or water

Combine mayonnaise, parsley, chives, lemon juice, dill weed, onion powder, salt and pepper in medium bowl; mix well. Stir in 1 tablespoon coconut milk; add additional milk, if desired, to thin dressing to desired consistency. Refrigerate at least 30 minutes to allow flavors to blend.

# HOMEMADE KETCHUP

Makes about 1½ cups

1 can (8 ounces) tomato sauce
1 can (6 ounces) tomato paste
¼ cup water
3 tablespoons maple syrup
2 tablespoons cider vinegar
¾ teaspoon salt

¼ teaspoon onion powder
¼ teaspoon garlic powder
¼ teaspoon ground mustard
¼ teaspoon ground cinnamon
Pinch ground allspice

Combine all ingredients in small saucepan; bring to a simmer over medium heat. Reduce heat to low; simmer 20 to 25 minutes or until thickened, stirring occasionally. Cool to room temperature; refrigerate up to 1 week.

## WHAT ABOUT SNACKS?

Think about cut-up fresh or roasted vegetables (such as Beet Chips, page 252), or delicious dips like salsa or Savory Pumpkin Hummus (page 260). If you have a sweet tooth, you can satisfy some of those cravings with fruit. Visit local farmers' markets for great selections—fruit will always taste best and be most nutritious when it is in season. Shopping there may be as close as we can get to hunting and gathering! Or you can try a Paleo smoothie (pages 294—313) for a refreshing all-natural treat. Keep in mind that fruits contain fructose, which is sugar, and some can be high in carbs, so adjust your meals accordingly. Be careful of concentrated carbs and sugars in dried fruits and check ingredient lists for hidden sugars.

## MAKE PALEO FIT YOUR LIFE AND ENJOY WHAT YOU EAT

A healthy diet is one you can stick with for life and that can be tailored to your tastes and sensitivities. Eating Paleo doesn't require counting calories or carbs. How many meals or snacks you have is up to you. Don't sweat it if you break the rules from time to time. This is not a crash diet. Eat whole, natural foods and enjoy them. If you can't live without cheese or the occasional slice of bread, add them in moderation. Once you experience how good it feels to eat the way evolution intended, the rest is easy!

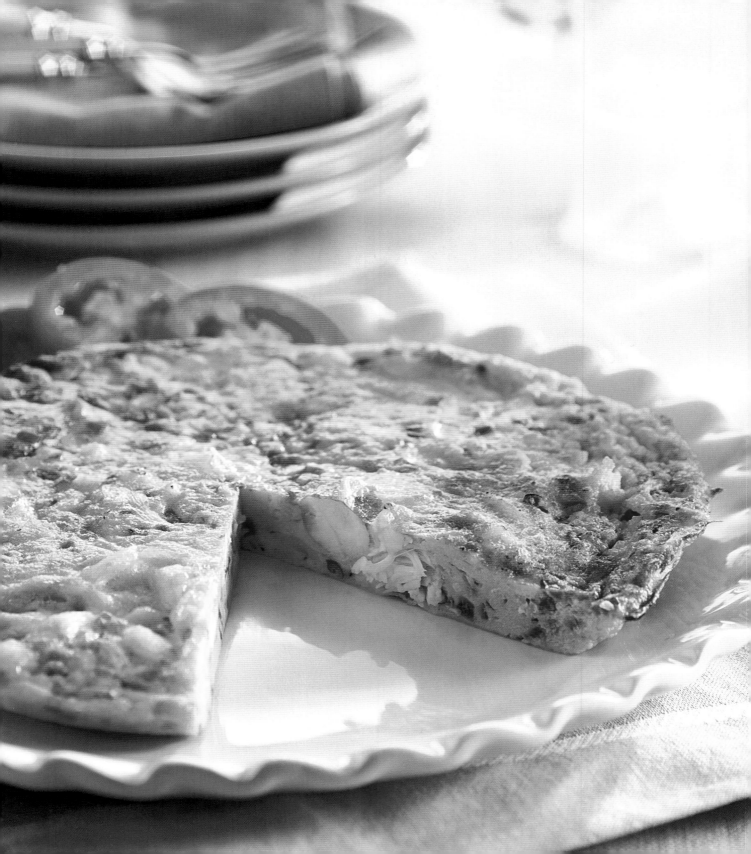

# EGGS

## SPICY CRABMEAT FRITTATA

Makes 4 servings

1 can (about
  6 ounces) lump
  white crabmeat,
  drained

6 eggs

¼ teaspoon salt

¼ teaspoon black
  pepper

¼ teaspoon hot
  pepper sauce

1 tablespoon olive oil

1 green bell pepper,
  finely chopped

2 cloves garlic, minced

1 plum tomato, seeded
  and finely chopped

**1.** Preheat broiler. Pick out and discard any shell or cartilage from crabmeat; break up large pieces of crabmeat.

**2.** Beat eggs in medium bowl. Add crabmeat, salt, black pepper and hot pepper sauce; mix well.

**3.** Heat oil in large ovenproof nonstick skillet over medium-high heat. Add bell pepper and garlic; cook and stir 3 minutes or until softened. Add tomato; cook and stir 1 minute. Stir in egg mixture; cook over medium-low heat 7 minutes or until eggs begin to set around edge of skillet, lifting edge with spatula to allow uncooked portion to flow underneath.

**4.** Transfer skillet to oven; broil 4 inches from heat source 1 to 2 minutes or until golden brown and center is set.

# BACON AND EGG CUPS

Makes 12 servings

1 tablespoon olive oil, plus additional for pan

12 slices bacon, crisp-cooked and cut crosswise into thirds

½ cup diced onion

½ cup diced red and green bell pepper

6 eggs

¼ cup canned coconut milk, well shaken

½ teaspoon salt

¼ teaspoon black pepper

**1.** Preheat oven to 350°F. Coat 12 standard (2½-inch) muffin cups with oil (or use bacon drippings). Place 3 bacon slices in each prepared muffin cup, overlapping in bottom.

**2.** Heat 1 tablespoon oil in medium skillet over medium-high heat. Add onion and bell pepper; cook and stir about 5 minutes or until vegetables are softened. Set aside to cool slightly.

**3.** Beat eggs, coconut milk, salt and black pepper in medium bowl until well blended. Stir in onion mixture until blended. Fill each muffin cup with scant ¼ cup egg mixture.

**4.** Bake 18 to 20 minutes or until eggs are set in center. Loosen sides with small spatula or knife; remove to wire rack. Serve warm.

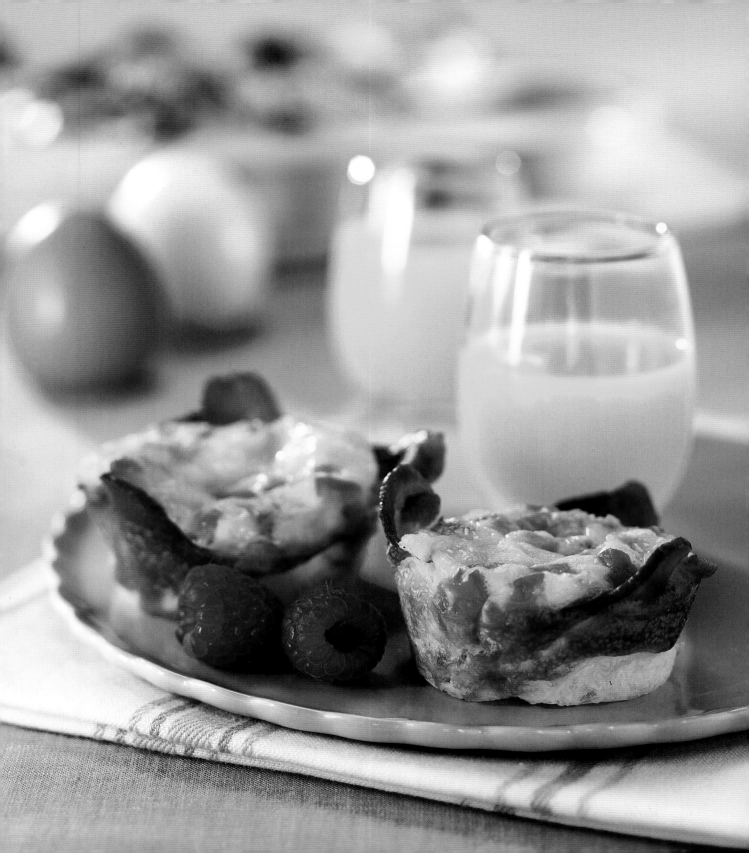

# SMOKED SALMON AND SPINACH FRITTATA

Makes 6 to 8 servings

2 tablespoons olive oil, divided

1 medium red onion, diced

1 clove garlic, minced

6 ounces baby spinach

10 eggs

1 teaspoon dried dill weed

¼ teaspoon salt

¼ teaspoon black pepper

4 ounces smoked salmon, chopped

**1.** Preheat broiler.

**2.** Heat 1 tablespoon oil in large ovenproof nonstick skillet. Add onion; cook 7 to 8 minutes or until softened, stirring occasionally. Add garlic; cook and stir 1 minute. Add spinach; cook and stir 3 minutes or just until wilted. Set aside to cool slightly.

**3.** Beat eggs, dill weed, salt and pepper in large bowl until blended. Stir in salmon and spinach mixture.

**4.** Heat remaining 1 tablespoon oil in same skillet over medium heat. Add egg mixture; cook about 3 minutes, stirring gently to form large curds. Cook without stirring 5 minutes or until eggs are just beginning to set.

**5.** Transfer skillet to oven; broil 2 to 3 minutes or until frittata is puffed, set and lightly browned. Let stand 5 minutes. Carefully slide frittata onto large plate or cutting board; cut into wedges.

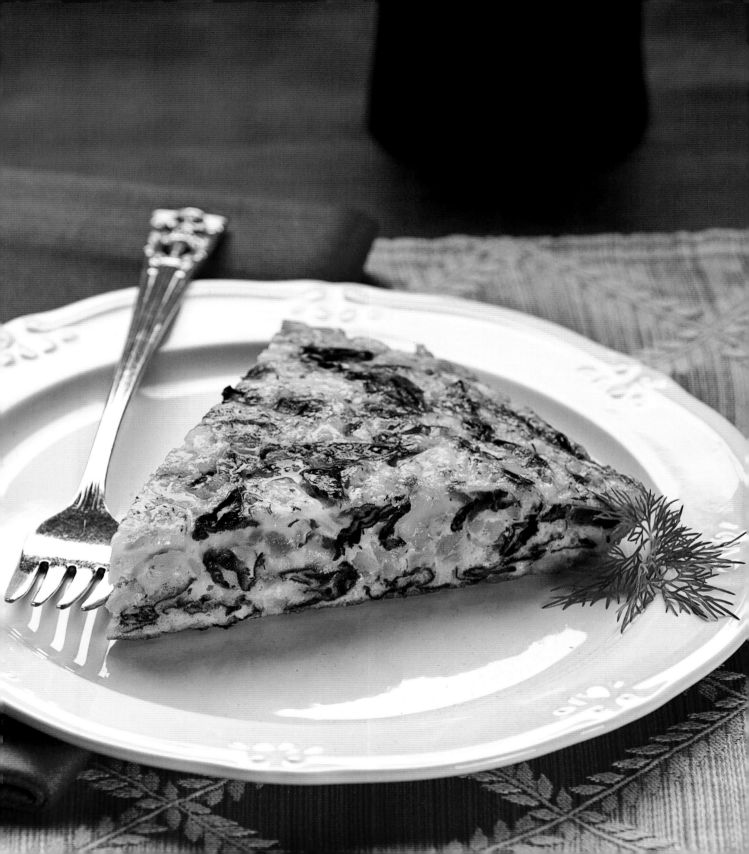

# EGGS RANCHEROS

Makes 4 servings

1 can (about 14 ounces) whole tomatoes, chopped, juice reserved

1 can (4 ounces) diced mild green chiles, drained

½ cup chopped onion

1 tablespoon white wine vinegar

¼ teaspoon salt

1 tablespoon olive oil

4 eggs

Salt and pepper to taste

**1.** Combine tomatoes with juice, chiles, onion, vinegar and salt in medium saucepan; cook over medium heat 20 minutes, stirring occasionally.

**2.** Heat oil in large skillet over medium-low heat. Break eggs into skillet; season with salt and pepper. Cook 2 to 3 minutes or until eggs are set. Turn eggs for over-easy eggs. Serve eggs with warm sauce.

# SCOTCH EGGS

Makes 6 servings

1½ to 2 tablespoons
  olive oil

1 pound ground beef
  or ground turkey

4 ounces bulk pork
  sausage

¼ teaspoon salt

⅛ teaspoon black
  pepper

6 hard-cooked eggs,
  peeled

**1.** Preheat oven to 400°F. Coat 11×7-inch baking dish lightly with oil.

**2.** Combine beef, sausage, salt and pepper in medium bowl; mix well. Divide mixture into six equal portions.

**3.** Coat hands lightly with oil. Working with one portion of meat mixture at a time, flatten meat mixture in palm of hand. Place one hard-cooked egg on meat mixture; wrap meat completely around egg. Press meat while turning in hands to completely seal. Brush wrapped eggs with oil; place in prepared baking dish.

**4.** Bake 30 minutes or until meat is cooked through and begins to brown. Cool slightly; cut in half to serve.

# MEDITERRANEAN ARTICHOKE OMELET

## Makes 1 serving

2 eggs

1 tablespoon olive oil

3 cans (14 ounces each) artichoke bottoms packed in water, drained, diced

1 ounce (about 2 pieces) roasted red peppers, diced

½ teaspoon minced garlic

Salsa

**1.** Beat eggs in small bowl.

**2.** Heat oil in large nonstick skillet over medium-high heat. Add artichokes; cook and stir 2 to 3 minutes or until beginning to brown. Add roasted peppers; cook and stir 2 minutes or until liquid has evaporated. Add garlic; cook and stir 30 seconds. Remove to small plate.

**3.** Add eggs to skillet; cook 1 to 2 minutes or until almost set, lifting edge of omelet with spatula to allow uncooked portion to flow underneath.

**4.** Spoon artichoke mixture onto half of omelet; fold omelet over filling. Cook 2 minutes or until set. Serve with salsa.

**NOTE:** Raw eggs will turn green if combined with raw artichokes because of a chemical reaction between the two foods. Cooking the artichokes separately will prevent this from happening.

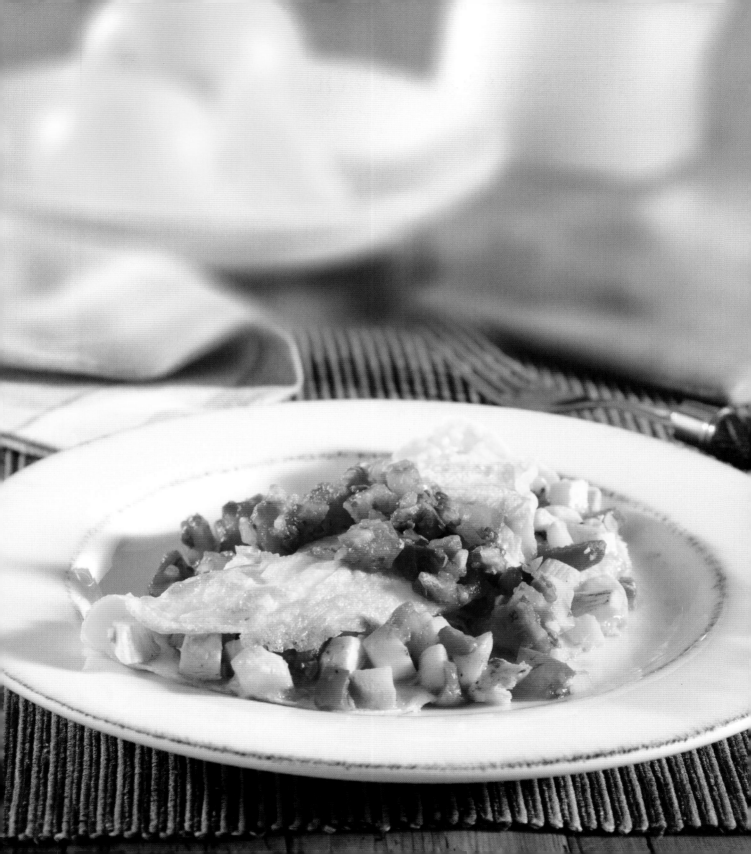

# MINI SPINACH FRITTATAS

## Makes 12 mini frittatas (4 to 6 servings)

1 tablespoon olive oil, plus additional for pan

½ cup chopped onion

10 eggs

¼ cup canned coconut milk, well shaken

1 package (10 ounces) frozen chopped spinach, thawed and squeezed dry

¾ teaspoon salt

⅛ teaspoon black pepper

⅛ teaspoon ground red pepper

Dash ground nutmeg

**1.** Preheat oven to 350°F. Generously coat 12 standard (2½-inch) muffin cups with oil.

**2.** Heat 1 tablespoon oil in medium skillet over medium heat. Add onion; cook and stir about 5 minutes or until tender. Set aside to cool slightly.

**3.** Beat eggs and coconut milk in large bowl until blended. Stir in spinach, onion, salt, black pepper, red pepper and nutmeg until well blended. Divide mixture evenly among prepared muffin cups.

**4.** Bake 18 to 20 minutes or until eggs are puffed and firm and no longer shiny. Cool in pan 2 minutes. Loosen bottom and sides with small spatula or knife; remove to wire rack. Serve warm, cold or at room temperature.

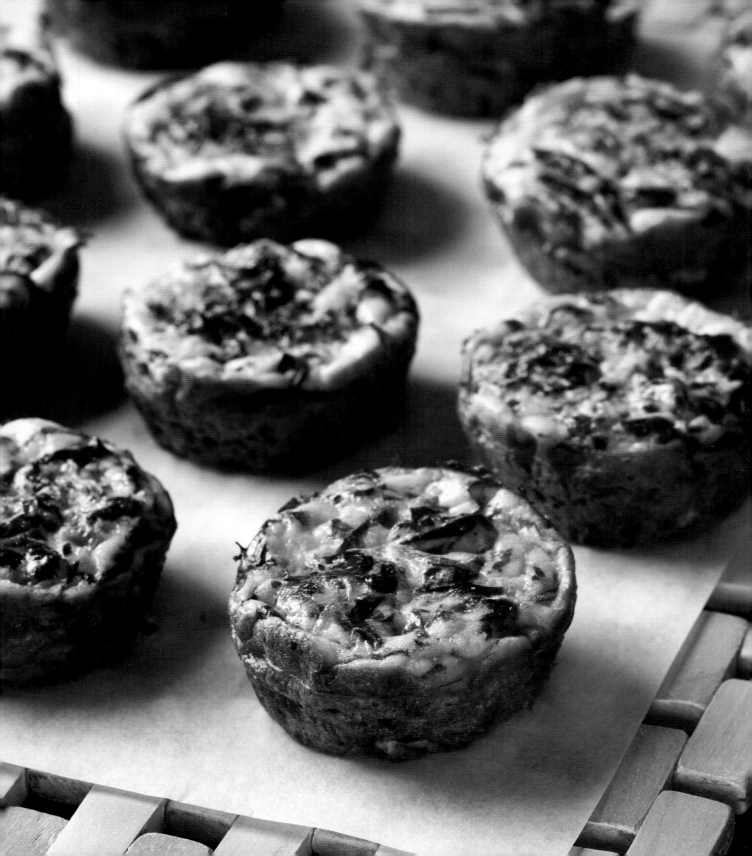

# CALIFORNIA OMELET WITH AVOCADO

Makes 4 servings

2 plum tomatoes, chopped

2 to 4 tablespoons chopped fresh cilantro

½ teaspoon salt, divided

8 eggs

1 tablespoon olive oil, divided

1 ripe medium avocado, diced

1 small cucumber, chopped

1 lemon, quartered

**1.** Preheat oven to 200°F. Combine tomatoes, cilantro and ¼ teaspoon salt in small bowl; mix well.

**2.** Beat eggs and remaining ¼ teaspoon salt in medium bowl until well blended.

**3.** Heat half of oil in small nonstick skillet over medium heat. Pour half of egg mixture into skillet; cook 2 minutes or until eggs begin to set. Lift edge of omelet with spatula to allow uncooked portion to flow underneath. Cook 3 minutes or until set.

**4.** Spoon half of tomato mixture onto half of omelet; fold omelet over filling. Slide omelet onto serving plate; keep warm in oven. Repeat with remaining oil, egg mixture and tomato mixture.

**5.** Cut omelets in half; top with avocado and cucumber. Serve with lemon wedges.

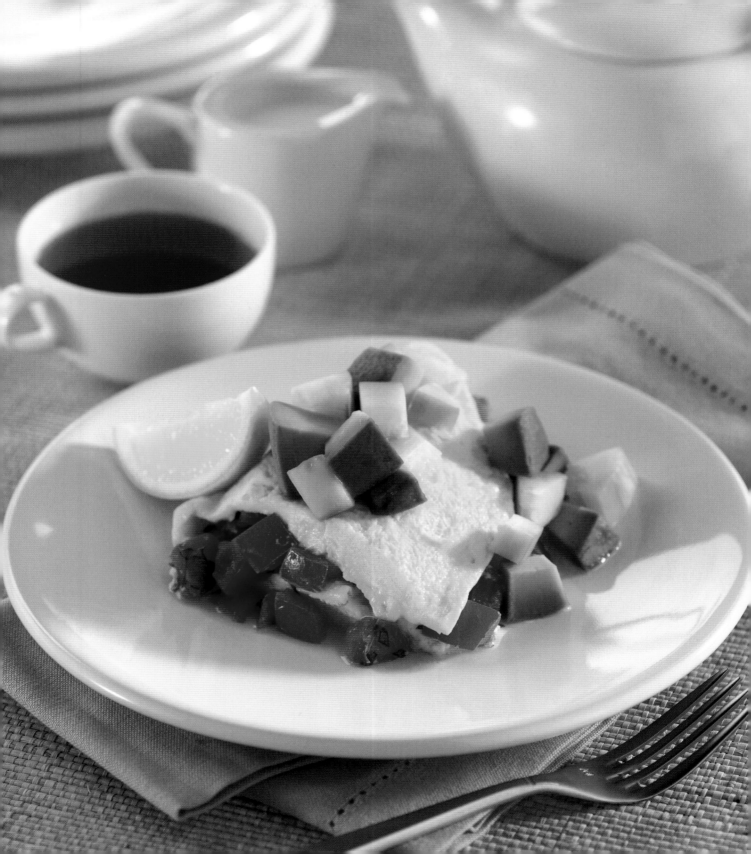

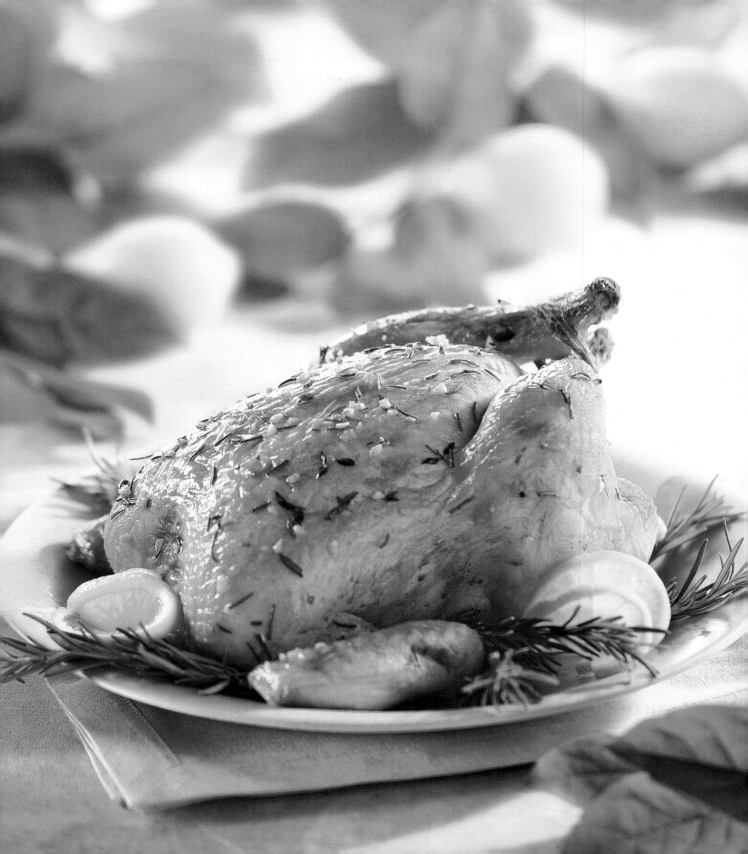

# POULTRY

## HERB ROASTED CHICKEN
Makes 4 servings

1 whole chicken (3 to 4 pounds)

1¼ teaspoons salt, divided

½ teaspoon black pepper, divided

1 lemon, cut into quarters

4 sprigs fresh rosemary, divided

4 sprigs fresh thyme, divided

4 cloves garlic, peeled

2 tablespoons olive oil

**1.** Preheat oven to 425°F. Place chicken, breast side up, in shallow roasting pan. Season cavity of chicken with ½ teaspoon salt and ¼ teaspoon pepper. Fill cavity with lemon quarters, 2 sprigs rosemary, 2 sprigs thyme and garlic cloves.

**2.** Chop remaining rosemary and thyme leaves; combine with oil, remaining ¾ teaspoon salt and ¼ teaspoon pepper in small bowl. Brush mixture over chicken.

**3.** Roast 30 minutes. *Reduce oven temperature to 375°F;* roast 35 to 45 minutes or until cooked through (165°F). Remove chicken to cutting board; tent with foil. Let stand 10 to 15 minutes before carving.

# GRILLED VIETNAMESE-STYLE CHICKEN WINGS

Makes 6 to 8 servings

3 pounds chicken wings

⅓ cup honey

¼ to ½ cup sliced lemongrass

¼ cup fish sauce

2 tablespoons chopped garlic

2 tablespoons chopped shallots

2 tablespoons chopped fresh ginger

2 tablespoons lime juice

2 tablespoons olive oil

Chopped fresh cilantro (optional)

Lime wedges (optional)

**1.** Remove and discard wing tips; cut each wing in half at joint. Place wings in large resealable food storage bag.

**2.** Combine honey, lemongrass, fish sauce, garlic, shallots, ginger, lime juice and oil in food processor; process until smooth. Pour marinade over wings. Seal bag; turn to coat. Marinate in refrigerator 4 hours or overnight.

**3.** Prepare grill for direct cooking or preheat grill pan. Preheat oven to 350°F. Line baking sheet with foil.

**4.** Remove wings from marinade; reserve marinade. Grill wings over medium heat 10 minutes or until browned, turning and basting occasionally with marinade. Discard remaining marinade.

**5.** Arrange wings in single layer on prepared baking sheet. Bake 20 minutes or until cooked through. Sprinkle with cilantro; serve with lime wedges, if desired.

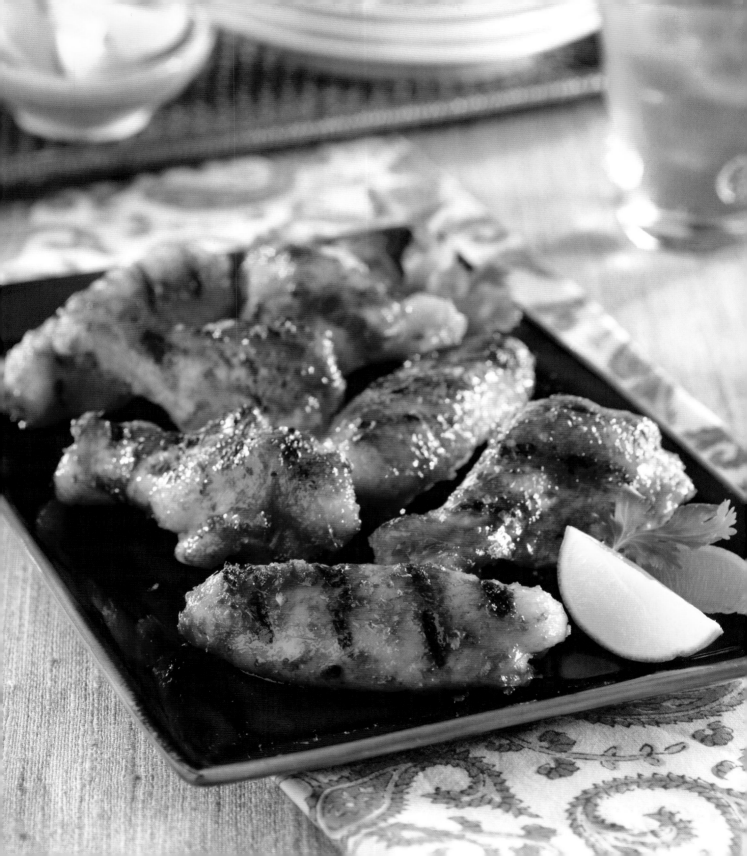

# BALSAMIC CHICKEN

Makes 6 servings

2 cloves garlic, minced

1½ teaspoons fresh rosemary leaves, minced *or* ½ teaspoon dried rosemary

¾ teaspoon black pepper

½ teaspoon salt

6 boneless skinless chicken breasts (4 to 6 ounces each)

1½ tablespoons olive oil, divided

¼ cup balsamic vinegar

**1.** Combine garlic, rosemary, pepper and salt in small bowl; mix well. Place chicken in large bowl; drizzle chicken with 1 tablespoon oil and rub with spice mixture. Cover and refrigerate 2 to 3 hours.

**2.** Preheat oven to 450°F. Brush shallow roasting pan or cast iron skillet with remaining ½ tablespoon oil. Place chicken in pan; roast 10 minutes. Turn chicken, stirring in 3 to 4 tablespoons water if drippings begin to stick to pan.

**3.** Roast about 10 minutes or until chicken is golden brown and no longer pink in center. If pan is dry, stir in 1 to 2 tablespoons water to loosen drippings.

**4.** Drizzle vinegar over chicken in pan. Transfer chicken to serving plates. Stir liquid in pan, scraping up browned bits. Drizzle over chicken.

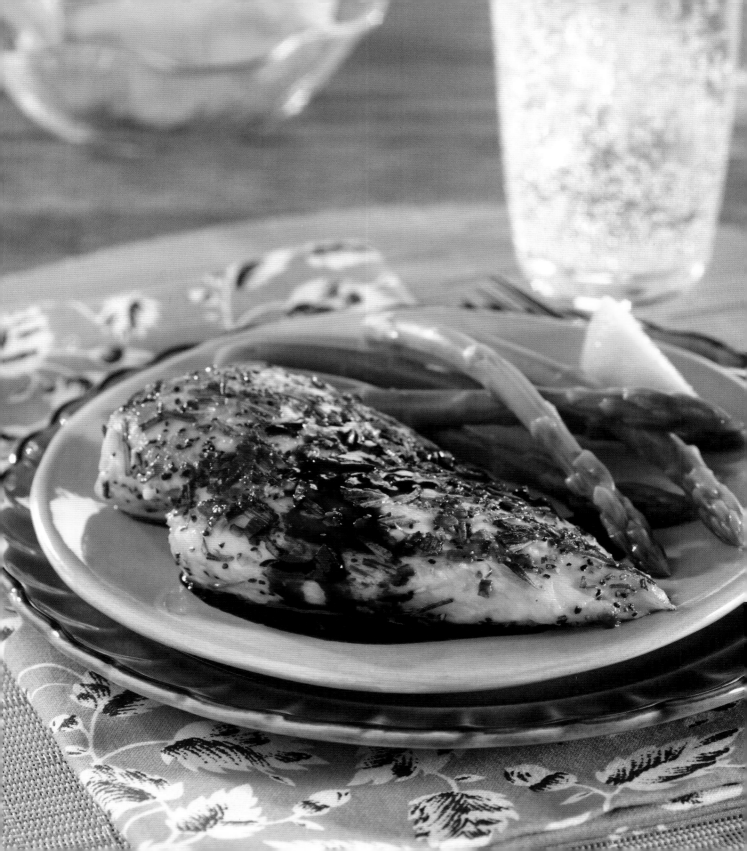

# JERK TURKEY STEW

Makes 4 servings

- 1 tablespoon olive oil
- 1 small red onion, chopped
- 1 clove garlic, minced
- ½ teaspoon salt
- ½ teaspoon ground ginger
- ¼ teaspoon black pepper
- ⅛ to ¼ teaspoon ground red pepper
- ⅛ teaspoon ground allspice
- 1 can (28 ounces) diced tomatoes
- 3 cups diced cooked turkey
- 2 cups diced cooked sweet potatoes (½-inch pieces)
- ½ cup chicken broth
- 1 tablespoon lime juice
- 1 tablespoon minced fresh chives

**1.** Heat oil in large saucepan or Dutch oven over medium heat. Add onion and garlic; cook and stir 5 minutes. Add salt, ginger, black pepper, red pepper and allspice; cook and stir 30 seconds.

**2.** Stir in tomatoes, turkey, sweet potatoes and broth; bring to a boil over high heat. Reduce heat to low; cook 15 minutes, stirring occasionally.

**3.** Stir in lime juice; cover and let stand 10 minutes. Sprinkle with chives just before serving.

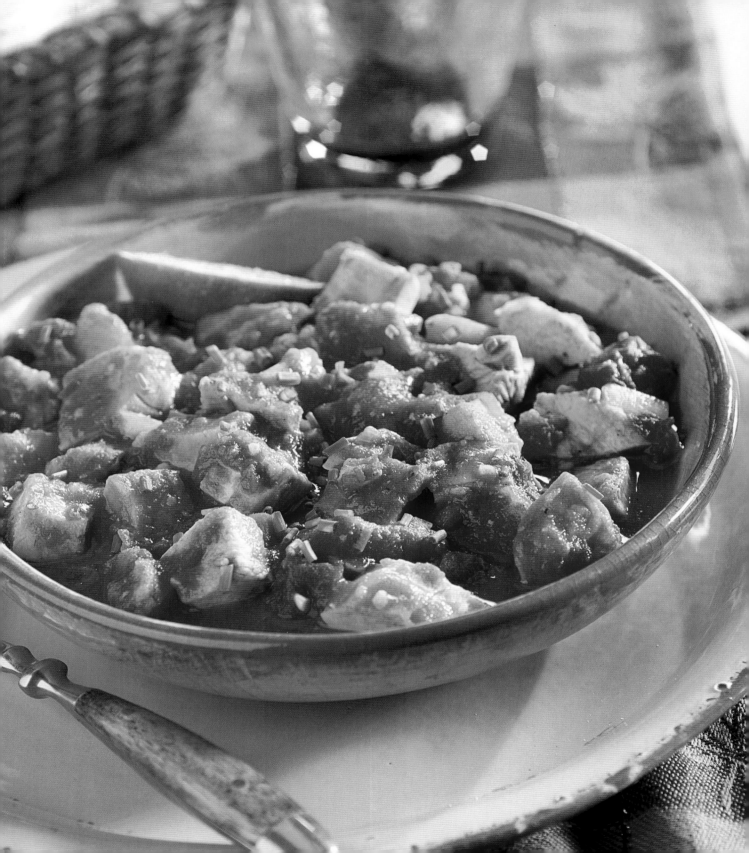

# SMOKED PAPRIKA DRUMSTICKS WITH SWEET POTATOES

Makes 2 to 4 servings

2 teaspoons smoked paprika

1 teaspoon garlic powder

1 teaspoon ground cumin

¾ teaspoon black pepper

½ teaspoon salt

4 (4-ounce) or 8 (2-ounce) chicken drumsticks, skin removed

12 ounces sweet potatoes, peeled and cut into 1-inch pieces

1 medium onion, cut into 8 wedges

1 tablespoon olive oil

**1.** Preheat oven to 350°F. Line baking sheet with foil.

**2.** Combine paprika, garlic powder, cumin, pepper and salt in small bowl; mix well. Coat chicken with spice mixture; place on prepared baking sheet.

**3.** Combine sweet potatoes, onion and oil in medium bowl; toss to coat. Arrange vegetables around chicken in single layer, leaving space between pieces.

**4.** Roast 30 minutes. Stir vegetables and turn chicken; roast 20 minutes or until chicken is cooked through (165°F).

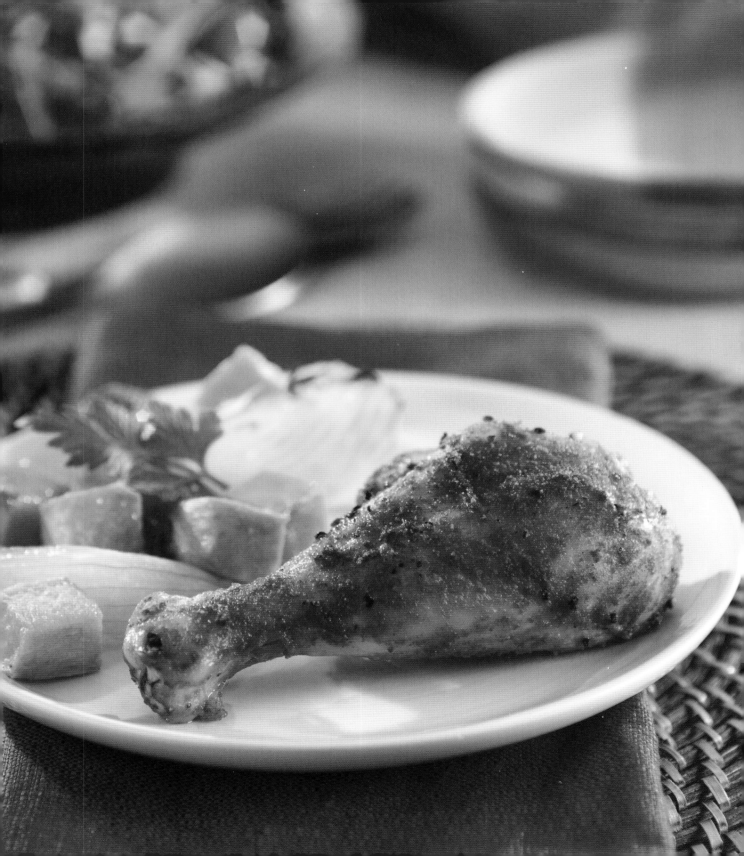

# POLLO DIAVOLO (DEVILED CHICKEN)

Makes 4 to 6 servings

8 bone-in skinless chicken thighs (2½ to 3 pounds)

¼ cup olive oil

3 tablespoons lemon juice

6 cloves garlic, minced

1 to 2 teaspoons red pepper flakes

1¼ teaspoons coarse salt, divided

3 tablespoons butter, softened

1 teaspoon dried sage

1 teaspoon dried thyme

¼ teaspoon ground red pepper or black pepper

Lemon wedges

**1.** Place chicken in large resealable food storage bag. Combine oil, lemon juice, garlic, red pepper flakes and ½ teaspoon salt in small bowl; mix well. Pour marinade over chicken. Seal bag; turn to coat. Marinate in refrigerator at least 1 hour or up to 8 hours, turning once.

**2.** Oil grid. Prepare grill for direct cooking. Drain chicken; reserve marinade.

**3.** Grill chicken, covered, over medium-high heat 8 minutes. Turn chicken; brush with reserved marinade. Discard remaining marinade. Grill, covered, 8 to 10 minutes or until chicken is cooked through (165°F).

**4.** Meanwhile, combine butter, sage, thyme, remaining ¾ teaspoon salt and ground red pepper in small bowl; mix well. Remove chicken to serving platter; spread herb butter over chicken. Serve with lemon wedges.

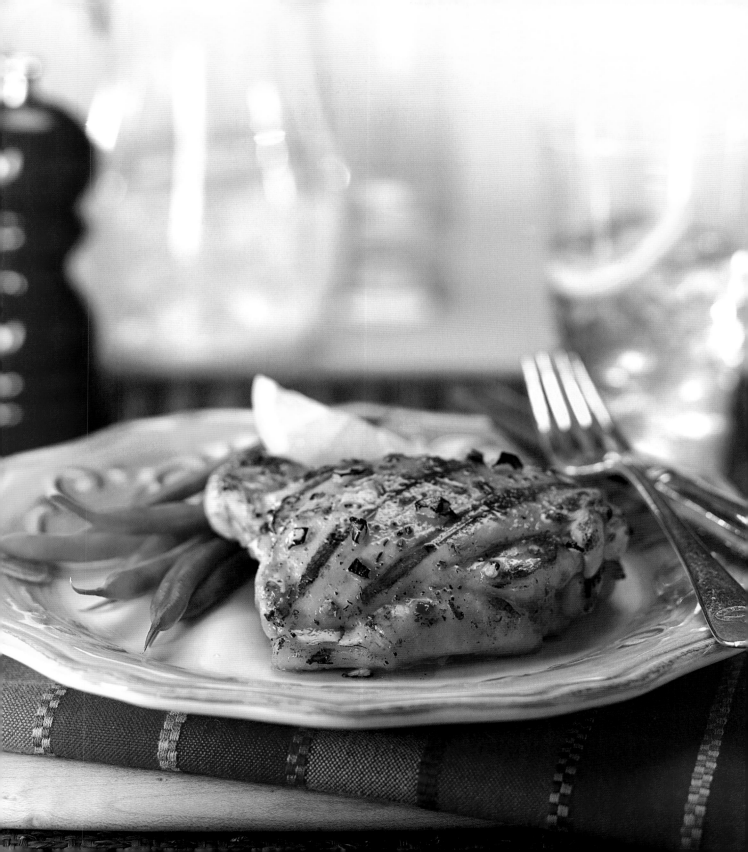

# SWEET SPICED TARRAGON ROAST TURKEY BREAST

Makes 4 servings

2 tablespoons olive oil, plus additional for pan

2 teaspoons grated orange peel

1½ teaspoons dried tarragon

1 teaspoon ground cumin

½ teaspoon salt

½ teaspoon ground ginger

½ teaspoon ground cinnamon

½ teaspoon ground allspice

½ teaspoon black pepper

¼ teaspoon ground red pepper

1 bone-in turkey breast (about 3 pounds)

**1.** Preheat oven to 400°F. Coat small roasting pan or baking sheet with oil.

**2.** Combine 2 tablespoons oil, orange peel, tarragon, cumin, salt, ginger, cinnamon, allspice, black pepper and red pepper in small bowl; mix well. Loosen skin from turkey; gently spread tarragon mixture under skin. Place turkey, skin side up, in prepared pan.

**3.** Roast 1 hour and 15 minutes or until turkey is cooked through (165°F). Remove to cutting board; tent with foil. Let stand 15 minutes before slicing.

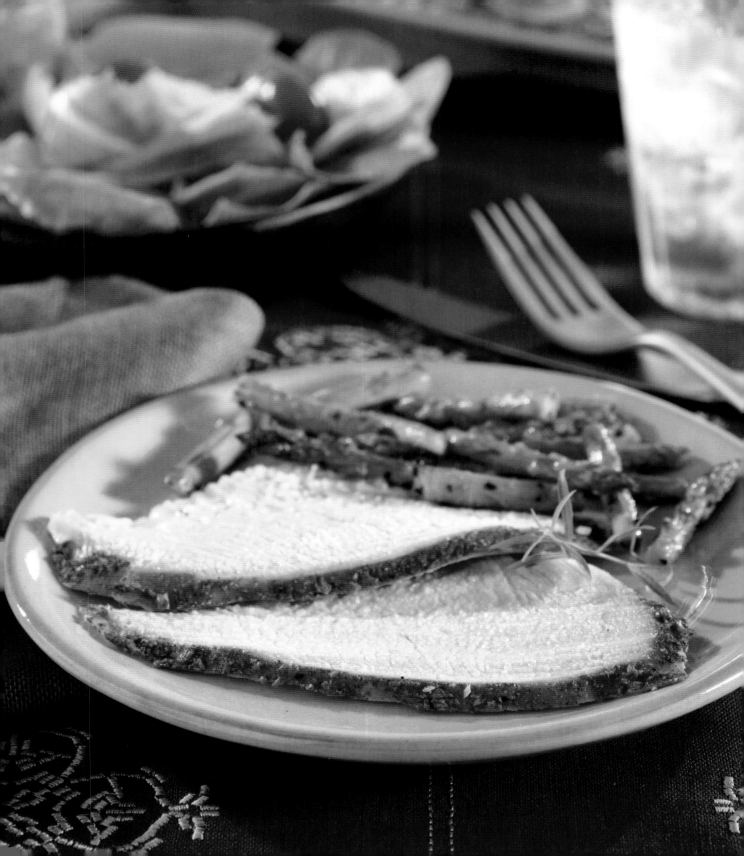

# SPICY SQUASH AND CHICKEN SOUP

Makes 4 servings

1 tablespoon coconut
  oil

1 small onion,
  finely chopped

1 stalk celery,
  finely chopped

2 cups chicken broth

2 cups cubed peeled
  butternut or
  delicata squash
  (about 1 small)

1 can (about
  14 ounces) diced
  tomatoes with
  green chiles

1 cup chopped
  cooked chicken

½ teaspoon salt

½ teaspoon
  ground ginger

⅛ teaspoon
  ground cumin

⅛ teaspoon
  black pepper

2 teaspoons lime juice

  Fresh parsley or
  cilantro sprigs
  (optional)

**1.** Heat oil in large saucepan over medium heat. Add onion and celery; cook and stir 5 minutes or until softened. Stir in broth, squash, tomatoes, chicken, salt, ginger, cumin and pepper; mix well.

**2.** Cover and cook over low heat 30 minutes or until squash is tender. Stir in lime juice; garnish with parsley.

**TIP:** Delicata and butternut are two types of winter squash with hard skins. Butternut is a long, light orange squash; delicata is an elongated, creamy yellow squash with green striations. To use, cut the squash lengthwise, scoop out the seeds, peel and cut into cubes.

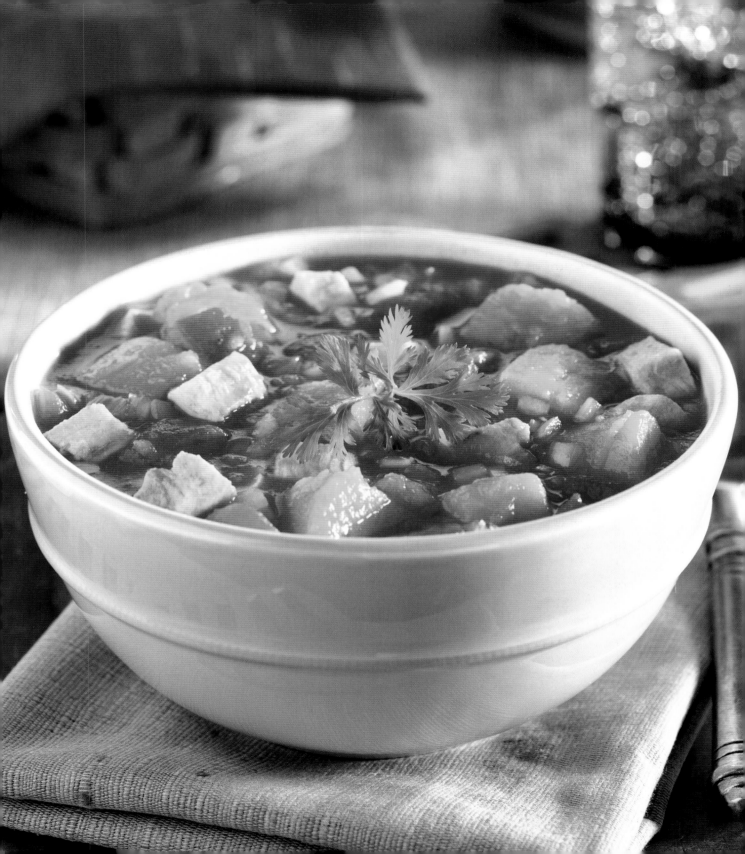

# GREEK LEMON CHICKEN

Makes 4 servings

4 boneless skinless
   chicken breasts
   (4 to 6 ounces each)

2 tablespoons olive oil,
   divided

2 tablespoons lemon
   juice

1 teaspoon grated
   lemon peel

1 clove garlic, minced

1 teaspoon
   dried oregano

½ teaspoon salt

⅛ teaspoon
   black pepper

Lemon wedges
   (optional)

Baby spinach
   (optional)

**1.** Place chicken in large resealable food storage bag. Add 1 tablespoon oil, lemon juice, lemon peel, garlic, oregano, salt and pepper. Seal bag; turn to coat. Marinate in refrigerator at least 30 minutes or up to 8 hours.

**2.** Heat remaining 1 tablespoon oil in large skillet over medium heat. Remove chicken from marinade; discard marinade. Add chicken to skillet; cook 3 minutes. Turn and cook over medium-low heat 7 minutes or until chicken is no longer pink in center. Serve with lemon wedges and spinach, if desired.

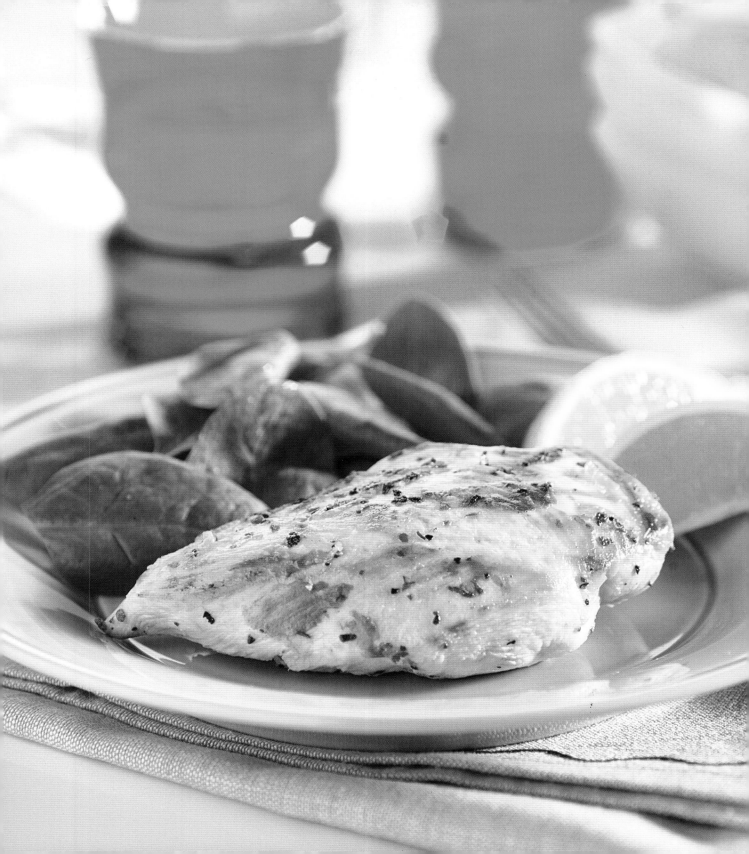

# FORTY-CLOVE CHICKEN FILICE

## Makes 4 to 6 servings

¼ cup olive oil

1 cut-up whole chicken (about 3 pounds)

40 cloves garlic (about 2 heads), peeled

4 stalks celery, thickly sliced

½ cup dry white wine

¼ cup dry vermouth

Grated peel and juice of 1 lemon

2 tablespoons finely chopped fresh parsley

2 teaspoons dried basil

1 teaspoon dried oregano

Pinch red pepper flakes

Salt and black pepper

**1.** Preheat oven to 375°F.

**2.** Heat oil in Dutch oven over medium-high heat. Add chicken; cook until browned on all sides.

**3.** Combine garlic, celery, wine, vermouth, lemon juice, lemon peel, parsley, basil, oregano and red pepper flakes in medium bowl; mix well. Pour over chicken; season with salt and black pepper.

**4.** Cover and bake 40 minutes. Uncover; bake 15 minutes or until chicken is cooked through (165°F).

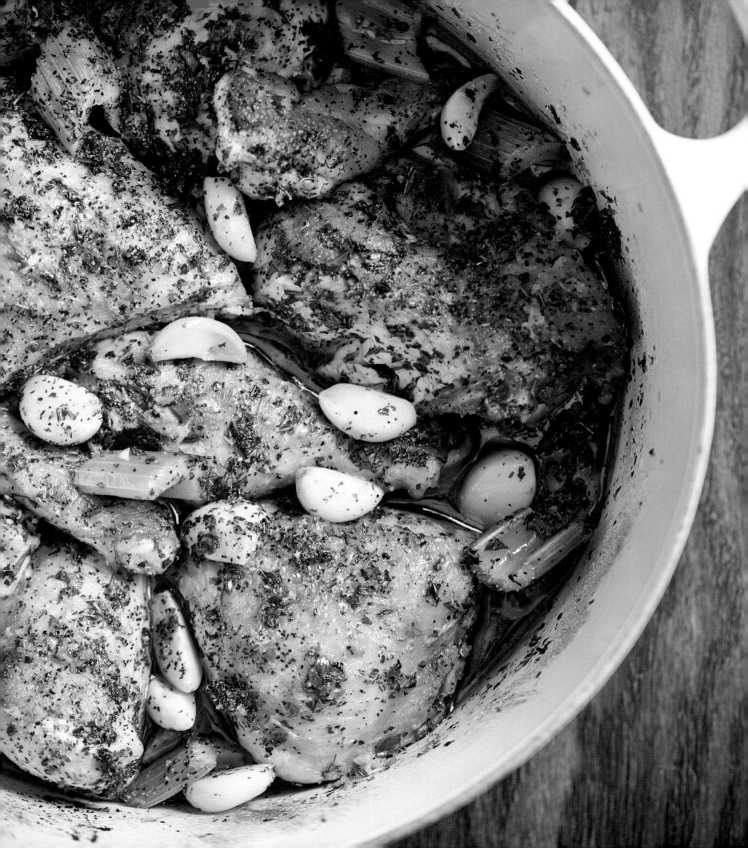

# HONEY-ROASTED CHICKEN AND BUTTERNUT SQUASH

Makes 4 to 6 servings

1 pound cubed peeled butternut squash

1 tablespoon plus 1 teaspoon olive oil, divided

Salt and black pepper

6 bone-in chicken thighs

1 tablespoon honey

**1.** Preheat oven to 375°F.

**2.** Place squash on large baking sheet. Drizzle with 1 tablespoon oil and season with salt and pepper; toss to coat. Spread in single layer on baking sheet.

**3.** Place wire rack over squash; brush rack with remaining 1 teaspoon oil. Arrange chicken on rack; season with salt and pepper.

**4.** Roast 25 minutes. Carefully lift rack and stir squash; brush honey over chicken. Roast 20 minutes or until squash is tender and chicken is cooked through (165°F).

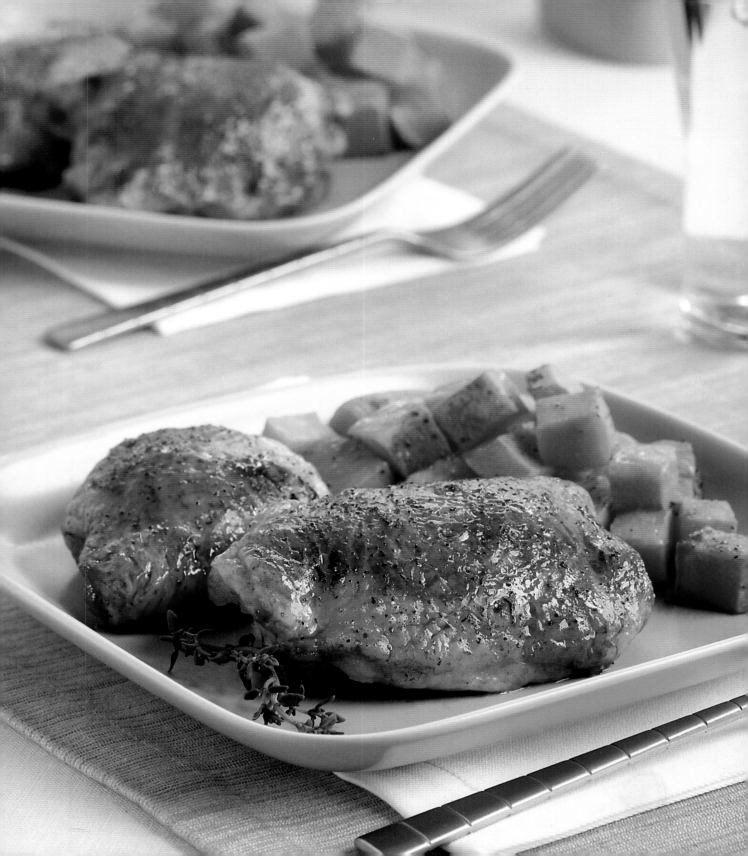

# GRILLED CHICKEN WITH CHIMICHURRI SALSA

Makes 4 servings

4 boneless skinless
  chicken breasts
  (4 to 6 ounces each)

½ cup plus 4 teaspoons
  olive oil, divided

  Salt and black pepper

½ cup finely chopped
  fresh parsley

¼ cup white wine
  vinegar

2 tablespoons finely
  chopped onion

3 cloves garlic, minced

1 fresh or canned
  jalapeño pepper,*
  finely chopped

2 teaspoons dried
  oregano

*Jalapeño peppers can sting and
irritate the skin, so wear rubber
gloves when handling peppers
and do not touch your eyes.*

**1.** Oil grid. Prepare grill for direct cooking.

**2.** Brush chicken with 4 teaspoons oil; season with salt and pepper.

**3.** Grill, covered, over medium heat 10 to 16 minutes or until chicken is no longer pink in center, turning once.

**4.** For salsa, combine remaining ½ cup oil, parsley, vinegar, onion, garlic, jalapeño and oregano in small bowl; mix well. Season with salt and pepper. Serve over chicken.

**TIP:** Chimichurri salsa is also good with grilled steak or fish. Store in an airtight container in the refrigerator for up to 24 hours.

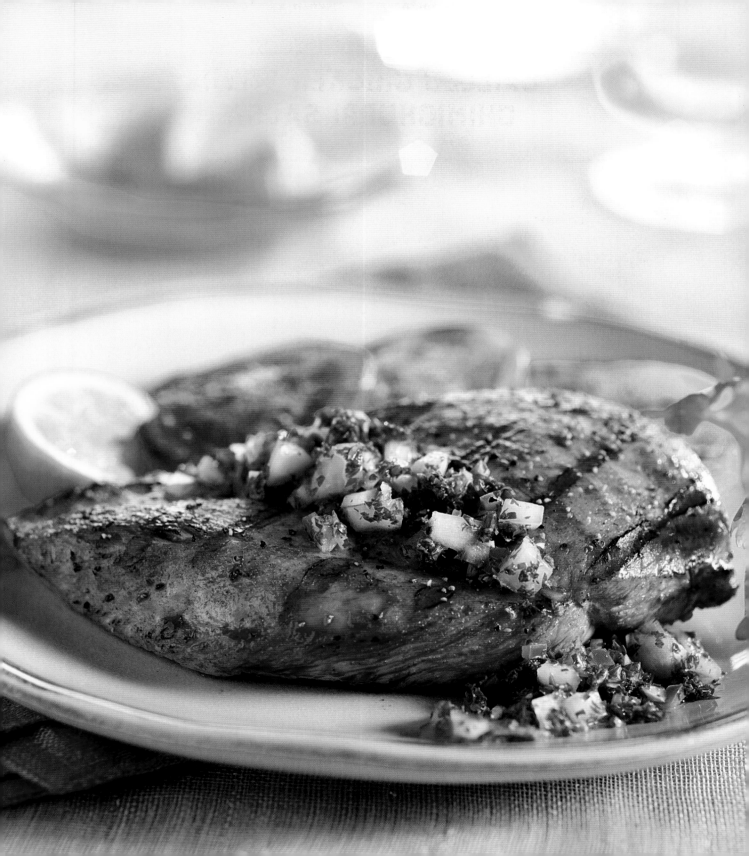

# SWEET POTATO AND TURKEY SAUSAGE HASH

Makes 2 servings

2 turkey Italian
   sausage links (about
   4 ounces each)

1 tablespoon olive oil

1 red onion, finely
   chopped

1 red bell pepper,
   finely chopped

1 sweet potato,
   peeled and cut
   into ½-inch cubes

½ teaspoon salt

¼ teaspoon
   black pepper

¼ teaspoon
   ground cumin

⅛ teaspoon chipotle
   chili powder

**1.** Remove sausage from casings; shape sausage into ½-inch balls.

**2.** Heat oil in large skillet over medium heat. Add sausage; cook 3 to 5 minutes or until browned, stirring occasionally. Remove to plate.

**3.** Add onion, bell pepper, sweet potato, salt, black pepper, cumin and chili powder to skillet; cook and stir 5 to 8 minutes or until sweet potato is tender.

**4.** Return sausage to skillet; cook without stirring 5 minutes or until hash is lightly browned.

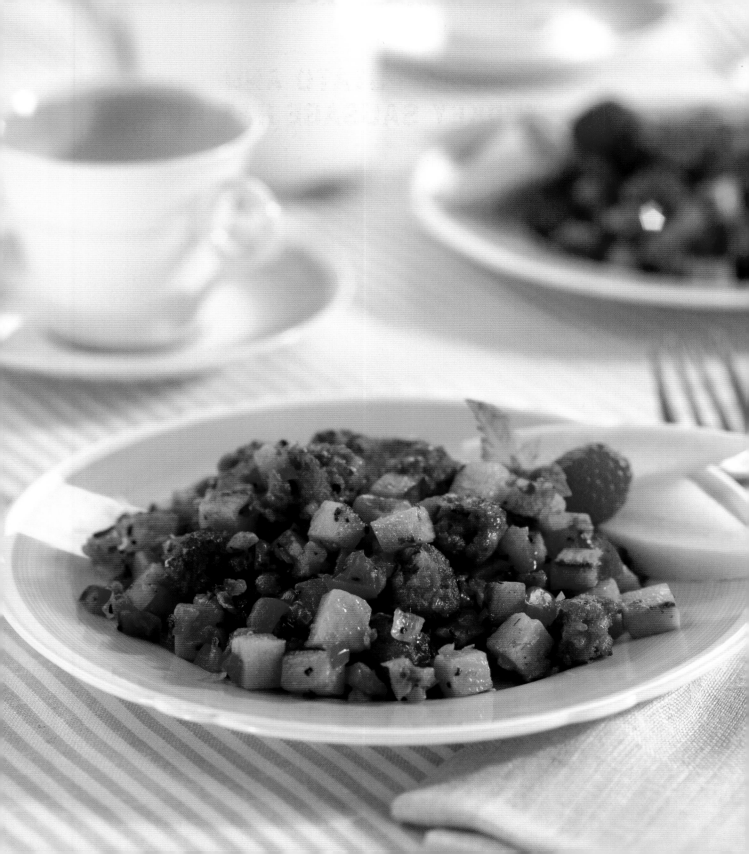

# ROAST CHICKEN WITH PEPPERS

Makes 6 servings

1 cut-up whole chicken (3 to 3½ pounds)

3 tablespoons olive oil, divided

1½ tablespoons chopped fresh rosemary leaves *or* 1½ teaspoons dried rosemary

1 tablespoon lemon juice

1¼ teaspoons salt, divided

¾ teaspoon black pepper, divided

3 bell peppers (red, yellow and/or green)

1 medium onion

**1.** Preheat oven to 375°F. Place chicken in shallow roasting pan.

**2.** Combine 2 tablespoons oil, rosemary and lemon juice in small bowl; mix well. Brush mixture over chicken; sprinkle with 1 teaspoon salt and ½ teaspoon black pepper. Roast 15 minutes.

**3.** Cut bell peppers into ½-inch strips. Cut onion into thin wedges. Combine vegetables, remaining 1 tablespoon oil, ¼ teaspoon salt and ¼ teaspoon pepper in medium bowl; toss to coat.

**4.** Arrange vegetables around chicken; roast about 50 minutes or until vegetables are tender and chicken is cooked through (165°F). Serve chicken with vegetables and pan juices.

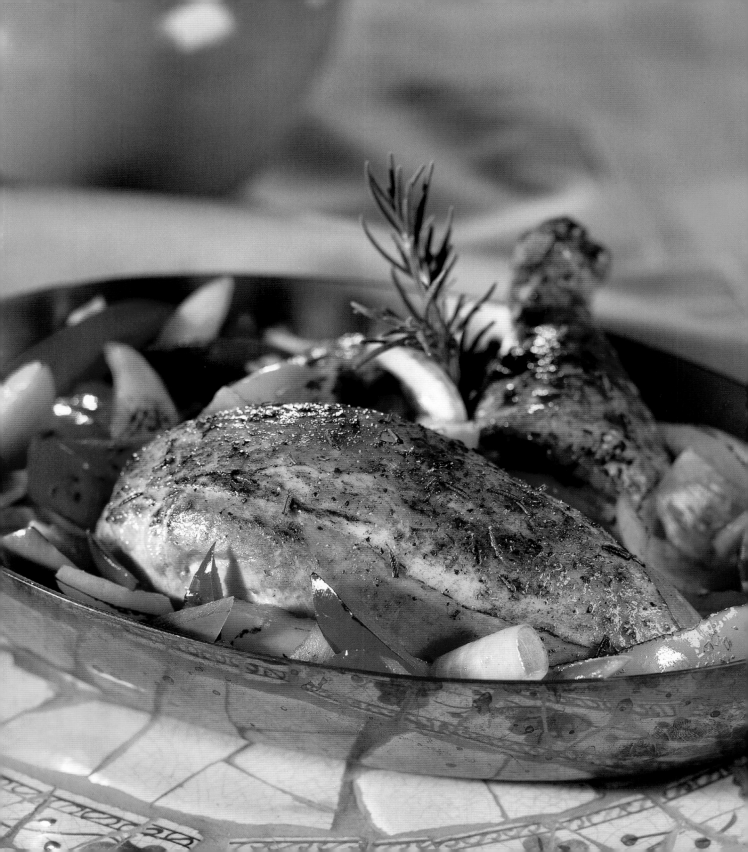

# GRILLED CHICKEN ADOBO

Makes 6 servings

½  cup chopped onion

⅓  cup lime juice

6  cloves garlic,
    coarsely chopped

1  teaspoon
    dried oregano

1  teaspoon
    ground cumin

½  teaspoon
    dried thyme

¼  teaspoon ground
    red pepper

6  boneless skinless
    chicken breasts
    (4 to 6 ounces each)

    Chopped fresh
    cilantro (optional)

**1.** Combine onion, lime juice and garlic in food processor; process until onion is finely minced. Transfer to large resealable food storage bag.

**2.** Add oregano, cumin, thyme and red pepper; knead bag until blended. Add chicken to bag. Seal bag; turn to coat. Marinate in refrigerator 30 minutes or up to 4 hours, turning occasionally.

**3.** Oil grid. Prepare grill for direct cooking. Remove chicken from marinade; discard marinade.

**4.** Grill chicken over medium heat 5 to 7 minutes per side or until no longer pink in center. Garnish with cilantro.

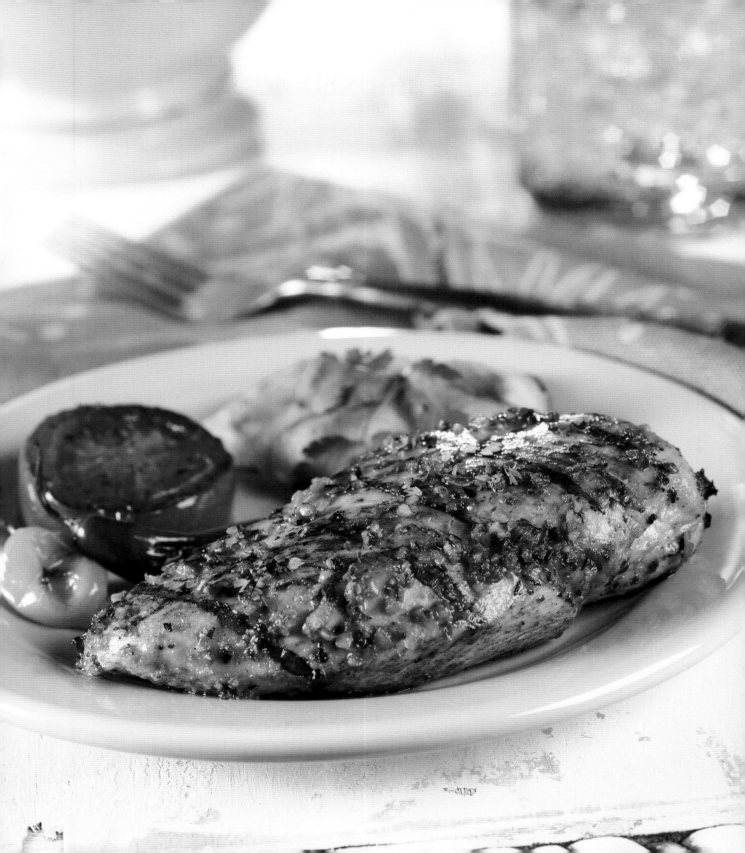

# CHUNKY CHICKEN STEW

Makes 2 servings

1 tablespoon olive oil

1 small onion, chopped

1 cup thinly sliced carrots

1 cup chicken broth

1 clove garlic, minced

½ teaspoon salt

⅛ teaspoon black pepper

1 can (about 14 ounces) diced tomatoes

1 cup diced cooked chicken breast

3 cups sliced kale or baby spinach

**1.** Heat oil in large saucepan over medium-high heat. Add onion; cook and stir 5 to 7 minutes or until golden brown. Stir in carrots, broth, garlic, salt and pepper; bring to a boil. Reduce heat to medium-low; cook, uncovered, 5 minutes.

**2.** Stir in tomatoes; cook 5 minutes or until carrots are tender. Add chicken; cook and stir until heated through. Add kale; cook and stir until wilted.

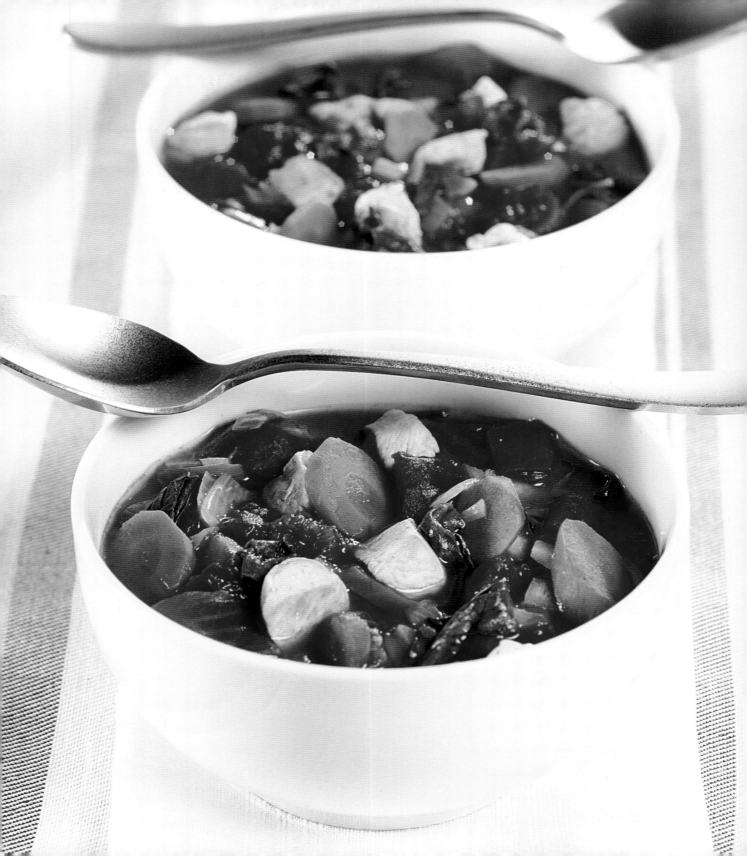

# TURKEY MEATBALLS WITH SPAGHETTI SQUASH

Makes 4 servings

1 tablespoon olive oil

1 egg

1 pound ground turkey

½ cup finely chopped onion

¼ cup almond flour

2 tablespoons chopped fresh parsley

1¼ teaspoons salt, divided

1 teaspoon garlic powder

¾ teaspoon dried thyme

¼ teaspoon fennel seeds

¼ teaspoon black pepper

⅛ teaspoon red pepper flakes

1 spaghetti squash (12 to 16 ounces)

¼ cup water

1 can (about 14 ounces) crushed tomatoes

¾ cup chicken broth

⅓ cup finely chopped green onions

½ teaspoon dried basil

½ teaspoon dried oregano

**1.** Preheat broiler. Line large baking sheet with foil; brush with oil.

**2.** Beat egg in large bowl. Add turkey, onion, almond flour, parsley, 1 teaspoon salt, garlic powder, thyme, fennel seeds, black pepper and red pepper flakes; mix well. Shape mixture into 20 meatballs; place on prepared baking sheet.

**3.** Broil meatballs 4 to 5 minutes or until tops are browned. Turn meatballs; broil 4 minutes.

**4.** Split squash in half and remove seeds. Place in glass baking dish, cut sides down; add water. Microwave on HIGH 10 to 12 minutes or until fork-tender. Set aside to cool.

**5.** Meanwhile, combine tomatoes, broth, green onions, basil, oregano and remaining ¼ teaspoon salt in large skillet; bring to a simmer over medium heat. Add meatballs; stir to coat. Reduce heat to medium-low; cook 10 minutes.

**6.** Scrape squash into strands into serving bowls or plates. Top with meatballs and sauce.

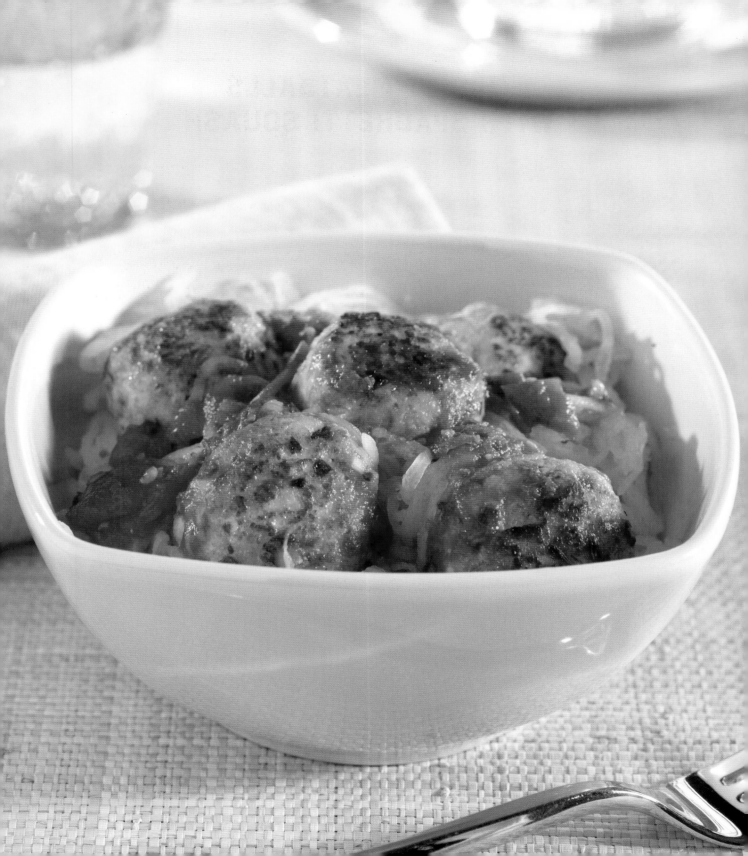

# CHICKEN PICCATA

Makes 4 servings

½ cup almond flour

¾ teaspoon salt

¼ teaspoon black pepper

4 boneless skinless chicken breasts (4 to 6 ounces each)

2 tablespoons olive oil, divided

1 tablespoon butter

1 small shallot, minced

2 cloves garlic, minced

¾ cup chicken broth

1½ tablespoons lemon juice

2 tablespoons chopped fresh Italian parsley

1 tablespoon capers, drained

**1.** Preheat oven to 200°F. Line small baking pan with foil. Combine almond flour, salt and pepper in shallow dish; mix well.

**2.** Pound chicken to ½-inch thickness between sheets of waxed paper with flat side of meat mallet or rolling pin. Coat chicken with flour mixture, shaking off excess.

**3.** Heat 1 tablespoon oil and butter in large skillet over medium-high heat. Add chicken; cook about 5 minutes per side or until no longer pink in center. Remove to prepared pan; place in oven to keep warm while preparing sauce.

**4.** Wipe out any dark bits of almond flour from skillet with paper towel. Add remaining 1 tablespoon oil, shallot and garlic to skillet; cook and stir over medium heat 1 minute. Stir in broth and lemon juice; cook about 4 minutes or until sauce is reduced by half. Stir in parsley and capers. Spoon sauce over chicken.

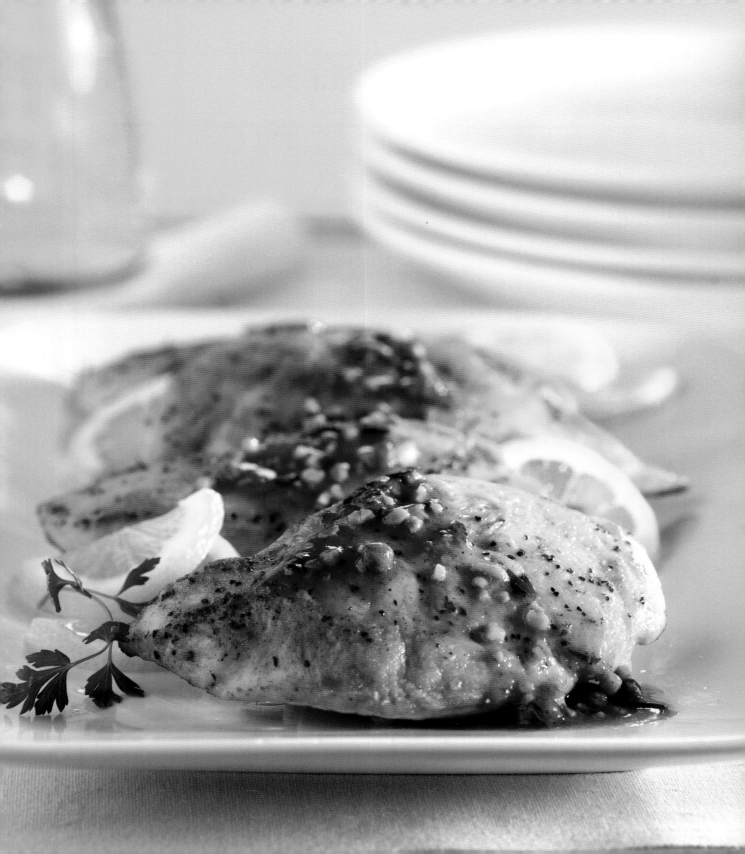

# CHICKEN SCARPIELLO

Makes 4 to 6 servings

3 tablespoons olive oil, divided

1 pound spicy Italian sausage, cut into 1-inch pieces

1 cut-up whole chicken* (about 3 pounds)

1 teaspoon salt, divided

1 large onion, chopped

2 red, yellow or orange bell peppers, cut into ¼-inch strips

3 cloves garlic, minced

½ cup dry white wine

½ cup chicken broth

½ cup coarsely chopped seeded hot cherry peppers

½ cup liquid from cherry pepper jar

1 teaspoon dried oregano

¼ teaspoon black pepper

¼ cup chopped fresh Italian parsley

*Or purchase 2 bone-in chicken leg quarters and 2 chicken breasts; separate drumsticks and thighs and cut breasts in half.

**1.** Heat 1 tablespoon oil in large skillet over medium-high heat. Add sausage; cook about 10 minutes or until well browned, stirring occasionally. Remove to plate.

**2.** Heat 1 tablespoon oil in same skillet. Sprinkle chicken with ½ teaspoon salt; arrange skin side down in single layer in skillet (cook in batches if necessary). Cook about 6 minutes per side or until browned. Remove to plate. Drain fat from skillet.

**3.** Heat remaining 1 tablespoon oil in skillet. Add onion and remaining ½ teaspoon salt; cook and stir 3 minutes or until softened, scraping up browned bits from bottom of skillet. Add bell peppers and garlic; cook and stir 5 minutes. Stir in wine; cook until liquid is reduced by half. Stir in broth, cherry peppers, cherry pepper liquid, oregano and black pepper; bring to a simmer.

**4.** Return sausage and chicken along with any accumulated juices to skillet. Partially cover skillet; cook over medium-low heat 10 minutes. Uncover; cook 15 minutes or until chicken is cooked through (165°F). Sprinkle with parsley.

**TIP:** If too much liquid remains in the skillet when the chicken is cooked through, remove the chicken and sausage and continue cooking the sauce to reduce it slightly.

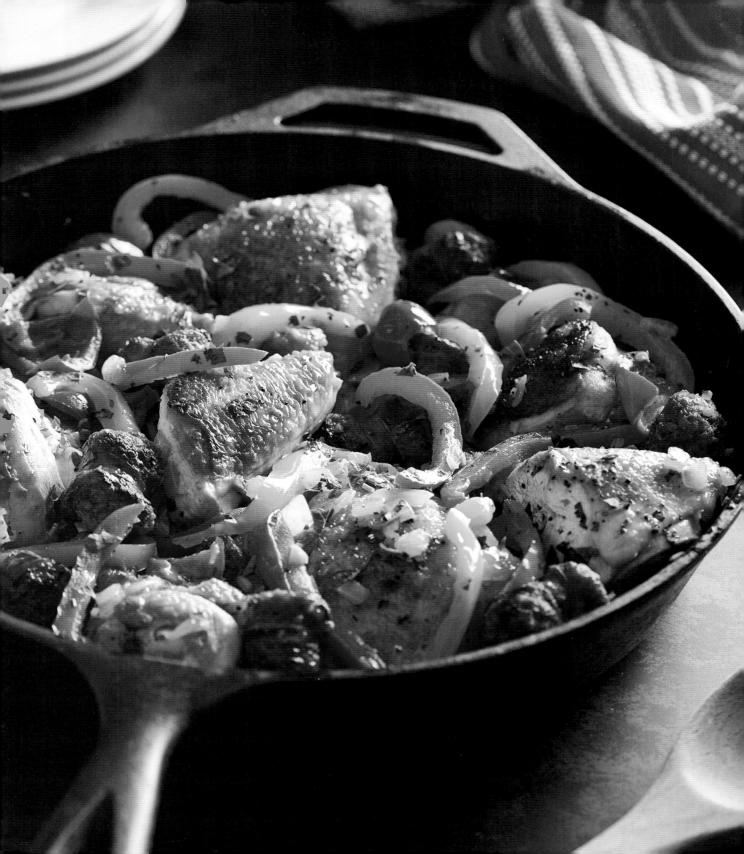

# CHILI ROASTED TURKEY WITH CILANTRO-LIME BUTTERNUT SQUASH

Makes 6 to 8 servings

## Turkey

Olive oil

1½ tablespoons chili powder

2 teaspoons dried oregano

1½ teaspoons ground cumin

½ teaspoon red pepper flakes

½ teaspoon salt

½ teaspoon black pepper

1 bone-in turkey breast (5 to 6 pounds)

## Squash

1 butternut squash, peeled, seeded and sliced

2 red bell peppers, cut into ¼-inch slices

2½ cups water

¾ teaspoon salt

½ teaspoon ground turmeric

1 cup chopped green onions

½ cup chopped fresh cilantro

3 tablespoons olive oil

2 to 3 tablespoons lime juice

1 tablespoon grated lime peel

**1.** Preheat oven to 325°F. Brush medium roasting pan and rack with oil. Combine chili powder, oregano, cumin, red pepper flakes, salt and black pepper in small bowl; mix well.

**2.** Loosen skin from turkey; gently spread spice mixture under skin. (If skin tears, use toothpick to hold skin together.) Place turkey, skin side up, on prepared rack in roasting pan.

**3.** Roast 1 hour and 30 minutes or until cooked through (165°F). Remove turkey to cutting board; tent with foil. Let stand 10 to 15 minutes before slicing. Remove and discard skin, if desired.

**4.** Meanwhile, place butternut squash in food processor; pulse until small pieces form.

**5.** Combine squash, bell peppers, water, salt and turmeric in large saucepan; bring to a boil over high heat. Reduce heat to low; cover and cook 10 minutes or until liquid has evaporated. Remove from heat; stir in green onions, cilantro, 3 tablespoons oil, lime juice and lime peel; mix well. Slice turkey; serve with squash mixture.

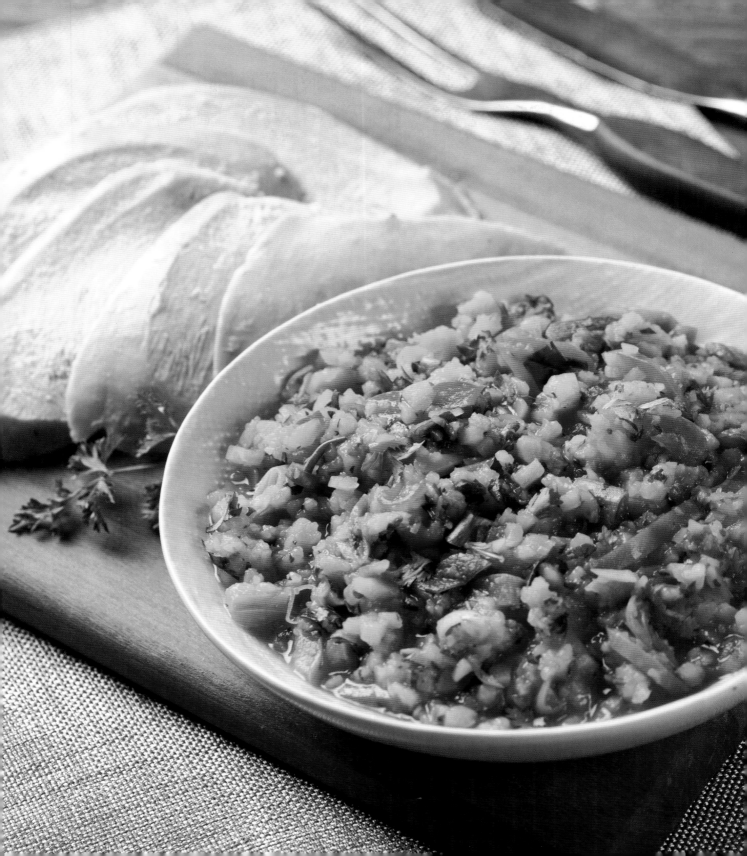

# PIQUANT CHICKEN WITH MUSHROOMS

Makes 4 servings

2 tablespoons olive oil, divided

4 boneless skinless chicken breasts (4 to 6 ounces each), pounded to ½-inch thickness

1 cup sliced mushrooms

½ cup dry white wine

Juice of 1 lemon

2 tablespoons capers

1 teaspoon chopped fresh dill, plus additional for garnish

½ teaspoon salt

Lemon wedges (optional)

**1.** Heat 1 tablespoon oil in large skillet over medium-high heat. Add chicken; cook 3 to 4 minutes or until beginning to brown.

**2.** Meanwhile, combine mushrooms, wine, lemon juice, capers, 1 teaspoon dill and salt in medium bowl; mix well.

**3.** Turn chicken, pour mushroom mixture over chicken. Reduce heat to medium-low; cover and cook 8 minutes or until chicken is no longer pink in center.

**4.** Remove chicken to serving platter; tent with foil. Cook liquid in skillet over medium-high heat 1 minute to reduce slightly. Remove from heat; stir in remaining 1 tablespoon oil. Pour sauce over chicken; garnish with additional dill and lemon wedges.

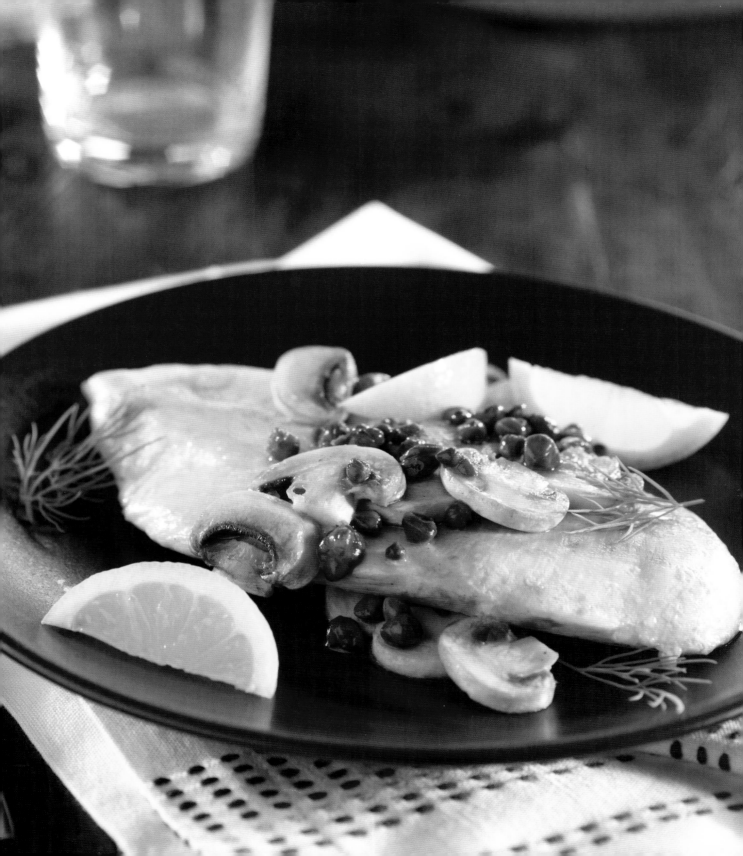

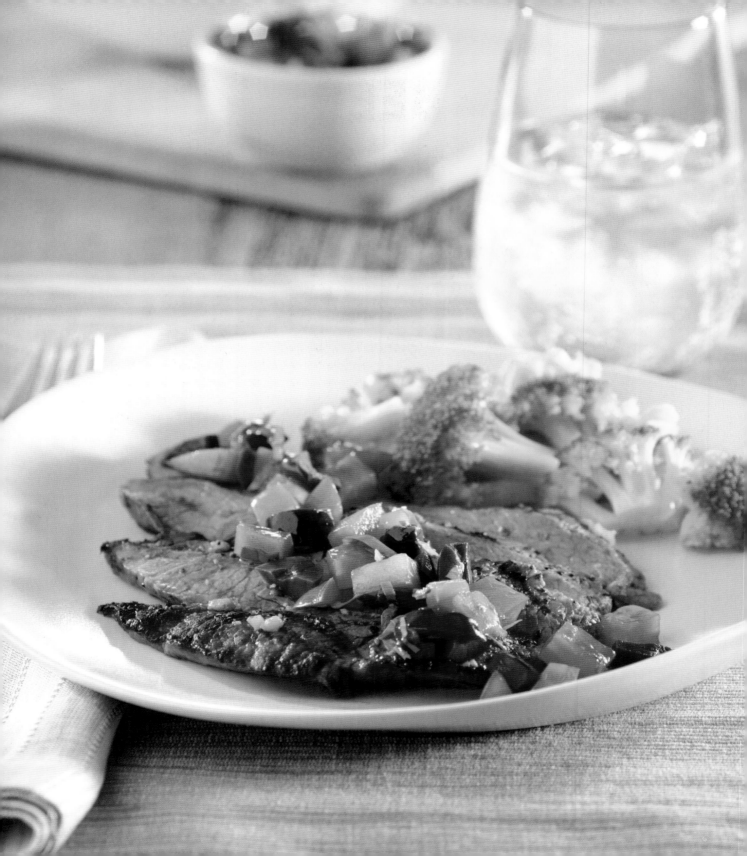

# BEEF

## FLANK STEAK WITH ITALIAN SALSA
### Makes 4 to 6 servings

2 tablespoons olive oil

2 teaspoons
balsamic vinegar

1 beef flank steak
(1½ pounds)

1 tablespoon
minced garlic

¾ teaspoon salt,
divided

¾ teaspoon black
pepper, divided

1 cup diced
plum tomatoes

⅓ cup chopped pitted
kalamata olives

2 tablespoons chopped
fresh basil

1. Whisk oil and vinegar in medium bowl until well blended. Place steak in shallow dish; spread garlic over both sides of steak. Sprinkle with ½ teaspoon salt and ½ teaspoon pepper; drizzle with 2 tablespoons oil mixture. (Reserve remaining mixture for salsa.) Cover and marinate steak in refrigerator at least 20 minutes or up to 2 hours.

2. Add tomatoes, olives, basil, remaining ¼ teaspoon salt and ¼ teaspoon pepper to oil mixture remaining in bowl; mix well.

3. Prepare grill for direct cooking or preheat broiler. Remove steak from marinade.

4. Grill steak over medium-high heat 5 to 6 minutes per side for medium rare or until desired doneness. Remove steak to cutting board; tent with foil. Let stand 5 minutes before slicing.

5. Cut steak diagonally across the grain into thin slices. Serve with tomato mixture.

# CHILI Á LA MEXICO

Makes 6 to 8 servings

2 pounds ground beef

2 cups finely chopped onions

2 cloves garlic, minced

1 can (28 ounces) whole tomatoes, coarsely chopped, juice reserved

1 can (6 ounces) tomato paste

1½ to 2 tablespoons chili powder

1 teaspoon ground cumin

¾ teaspoon salt

¼ teaspoon ground red pepper

¼ teaspoon ground cloves (optional)

Lime wedges

Fresh cilantro sprigs (optional)

**1.** Brown beef in deep skillet over medium-high heat 6 to 8 minutes, stirring to break up meat. Drain fat.

**2.** Add onions and garlic to skillet; cook and stir over medium heat 5 minutes or until onions are softened.

**3.** Stir in tomatoes with juice, tomato paste, chili powder, cumin, salt, red pepper and cloves, if desired; bring to a boil over high heat. Reduce heat to low; cover and cook 30 minutes, stirring occasionally. Serve with lime wedges; garnish with cilantro.

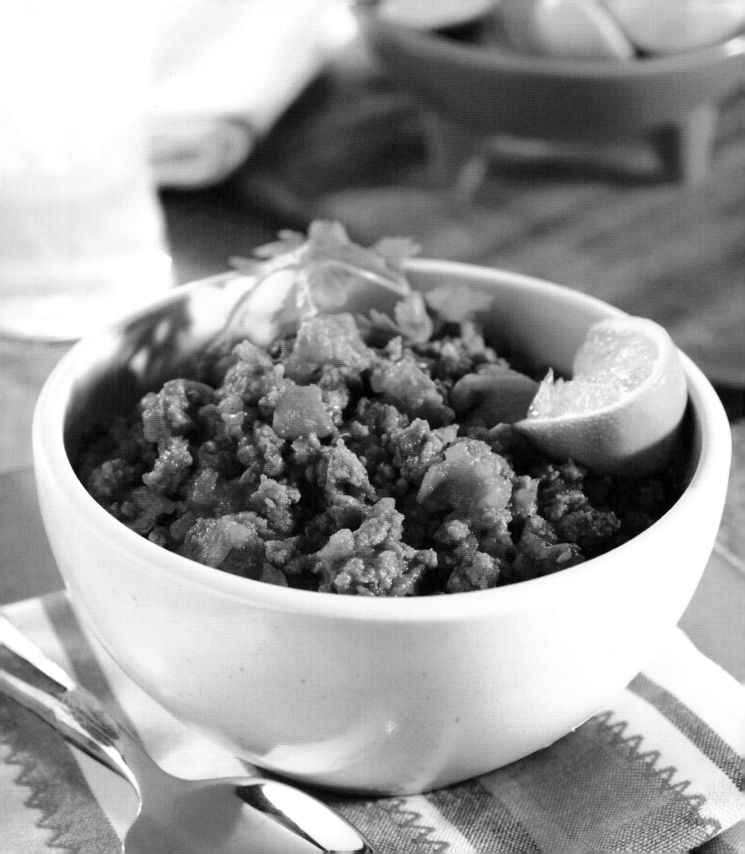

# TEXAS MEETS
# N.Y. STRIP STEAKS

Makes 4 servings

3 tablespoons olive oil, divided

2 medium onions, thinly sliced

¼ teaspoon coarse salt

4 strip steaks (6 to 8 ounces each)

2 teaspoons minced garlic

2 teaspoons black pepper

1. Heat 2 tablespoons oil in medium skillet over medium heat. Add onions; cook 15 to 20 minutes or until soft and golden brown, stirring occasionally. Stir in ¼ teaspoon salt.

2. Meanwhile, prepare grill for direct cooking. Rub steaks with remaining 1 tablespoon oil and garlic. Sprinkle pepper on both sides of steaks.

3. Grill steaks over medium-high heat 5 to 6 minutes per side until 145°F or until desired doneness. Season with additional salt; serve with onions.

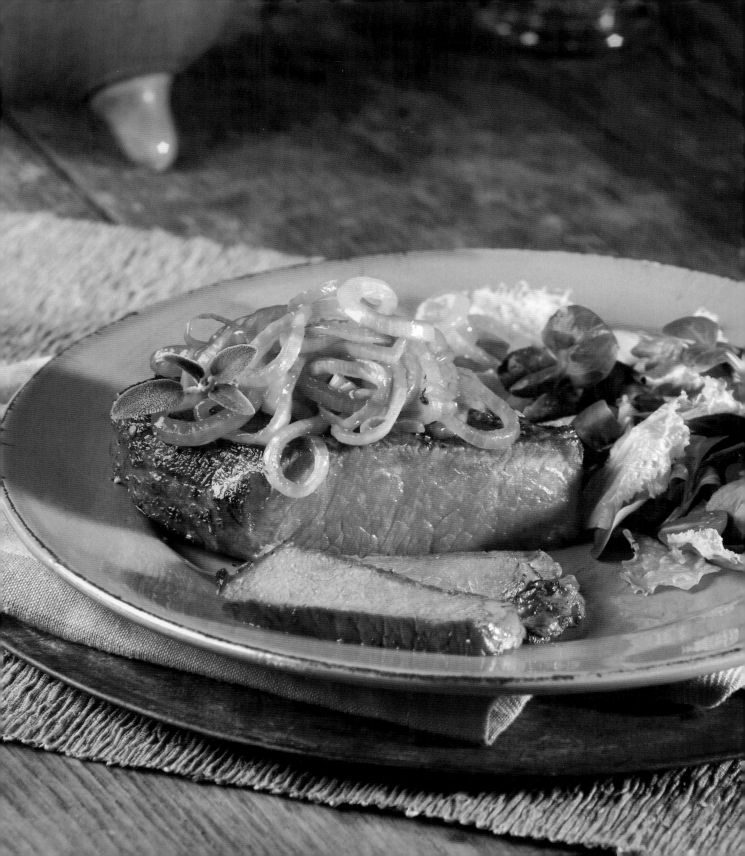

# RED WINE OREGANO BEEF KABOBS

Makes 4 servings

¼ cup dry red wine

¼ cup finely chopped
  fresh parsley

2 tablespoons Paleo
  Worcestershire
  Sauce (page 10)

1 tablespoon
  coconut aminos

3 cloves garlic, minced

1 teaspoon
  dried oregano

½ teaspoon salt

½ teaspoon
  black pepper

¾ pound boneless
  beef top sirloin
  steak, cut into
  16 (1-inch) pieces

16 whole mushrooms
  (about 8 ounces)

1 medium red onion,
  cut into eighths and
  layers separated

2 teaspoons olive oil

**1.** Combine wine, parsley, Worcestershire sauce, coconut aminos, garlic, oregano, salt and pepper in small bowl; mix well. Place steak, mushrooms and onion in large resealable food storage bag. Pour wine mixture over beef and vegetables. Seal bag; turn to coat. Marinate in refrigerator 1 hour, turning frequently.

**2.** Soak four 12-inch or eight 6-inch wooden skewers in water 20 minutes to prevent burning.

**3.** Preheat broiler. Brush broiler rack with oil. Alternately thread beef, mushrooms and onion onto skewers. Arrange skewers on prepared rack; brush with marinade.

**4.** Broil skewers 4 to 6 inches from heat source 8 to 10 minutes or until beef is tender, turning occasionally.

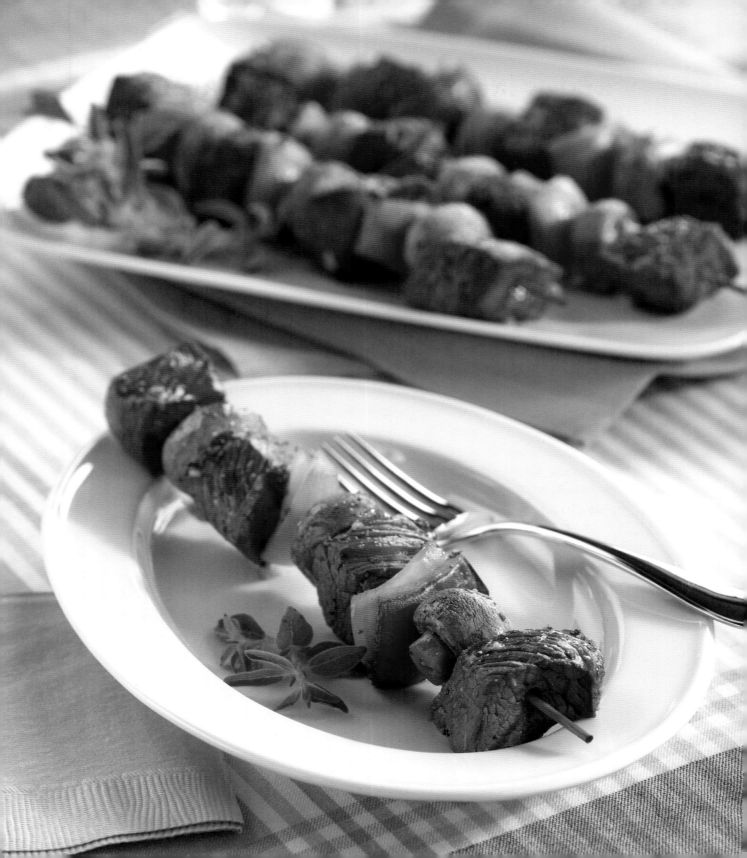

# SKIRT STEAK WITH RED PEPPER CHIMICHURRI

## Makes 4 servings

1½ tablespoons olive oil, plus additional for pan

1 clove garlic, peeled and cut in half

1 pound skirt steak, trimmed

¼ teaspoon salt

½ teaspoon black pepper, divided

1 cup diced roasted red pepper

1 shallot, minced

1 tablespoon capers

1 tablespoon white wine vinegar

1 clove garlic, minced

**1.** Preheat broiler. Brush broiler rack with oil. Rub steak on both sides with garlic clove; season with salt and ¼ teaspoon black pepper. Place on prepared rack.

**2.** Broil steak 4 inches from heat 4 to 5 minutes per side or until desired doneness. Remove steak to cutting board; tent with foil. Let stand 5 to 10 minutes before slicing.

**3.** Combine roasted peppers, 1½ tablespoons oil, shallot, capers, vinegar, minced garlic and remaining ¼ teaspoon black pepper in medium bowl; mix well.

**4.** Thinly slice steak against the grain; top with chimichurri sauce.

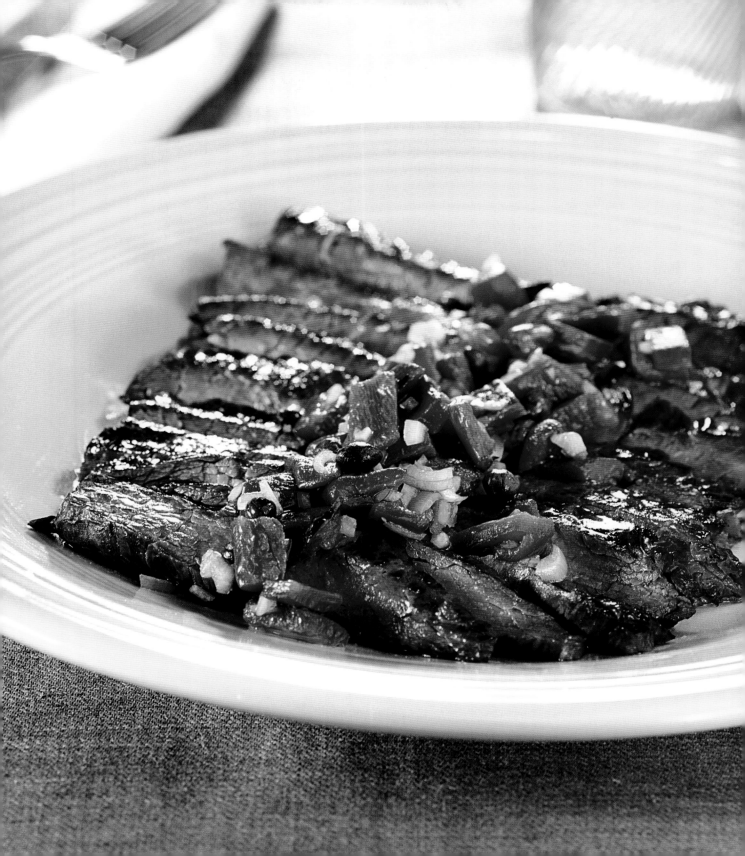

# LONDON BROIL WITH MARINATED VEGETABLES

### Makes 6 servings

¾ cup olive oil

¾ cup dry red wine

2 tablespoons
  red wine vinegar

2 tablespoons finely
  chopped shallots

2 teaspoons
  minced garlic

1 teaspoon salt

½ teaspoon
  dried thyme

½ teaspoon
  dried oregano

½ teaspoon dried basil

½ teaspoon
  black pepper

2 pounds top round
  London broil
  (1½ inches thick)

1 medium red onion,
  cut into ¼-inch-thick
  slices

1 package (8 ounces)
  sliced mushrooms

1 medium red bell
  pepper, cut into
  strips

1 medium zucchini,
  cut into ¼-inch-thick
  slices

**1.** Combine oil, wine, vinegar, shallots, garlic, salt, thyme, oregano, basil and black pepper in medium bowl; mix well. Place beef in large resealable food storage bag; pour ¾ cup marinade over beef. Seal bag; turn to coat. Marinate in refrigerator up to 24 hours, turning once or twice.

**2.** Combine onion, mushrooms, bell pepper, zucchini and remaining marinade in another large resealable food storage bag. Seal bag; turn to coat. Marinate in refrigerator up to 24 hours, turning once or twice.

**3.** Preheat broiler. Remove beef from marinade and place on broiler pan; discard marinade.

**4.** Broil 4 to 5 inches from heat about 9 minutes per side or until desired doneness. Remove beef to cutting board; tent with foil. Let stand 10 minutes before slicing.

**5.** Meanwhile, drain vegetables and arrange on broiler pan; discard marinade. Broil 4 to 5 inches from heat about 9 minutes or until edges of vegetables just begin to brown. Cut beef into thin slices; serve with vegetables.

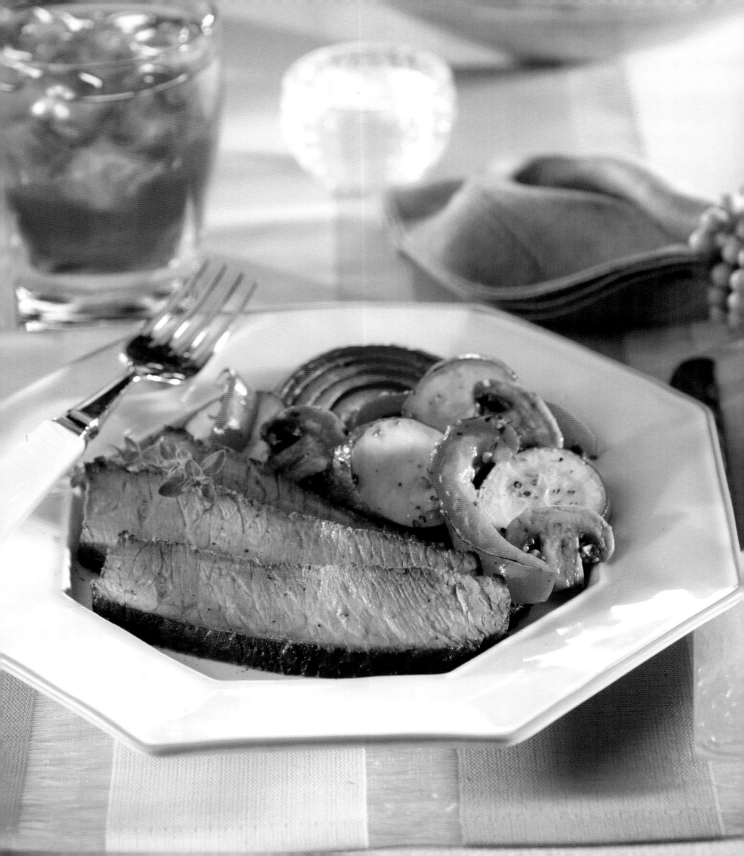

# BEEF TENDERLOIN WITH MERLOT SAUCE

Makes 6 servings

1½ tablespoons olive oil, divided

1 teaspoon garlic powder

1 teaspoon onion powder

¾ teaspoon salt, divided

½ teaspoon black pepper

1½ pounds beef tenderloin

⅔ cup merlot or other dry red wine

2 tablespoons balsamic vinegar

1 teaspoon honey

1. Preheat oven to 400°F. Coat 13×9-inch baking pan or baking sheet with ½ tablespoon oil. Combine garlic powder, onion powder, ½ teaspoon salt and pepper in small bowl; mix well. Sprinkle over top and sides of beef.

2. Heat remaining 1 tablespoon oil in large skillet over medium-high heat. Add beef; cook 4 minutes or until well browned. Turn and cook 4 minutes or until browned. Place beef in prepared pan (if necessary, tuck thinner end under for even cooking.)

3. Roast 27 to 32 minutes or until 135°F for medium rare or until desired doneness. Remove beef to cutting board; tent with foil. Let stand 10 minutes before slicing.

4. Meanwhile, return skillet with beef drippings to medium-high heat; stir in wine, vinegar, honey and remaining ¼ teaspoon salt. Bring to a boil, scraping up browned bits from bottom of skillet. Boil 1 to 2 minutes or until reduced to ⅓ cup.

5. Add any accumulated beef juices to merlot sauce in skillet, return to a boil. Slice beef; serve with sauce.

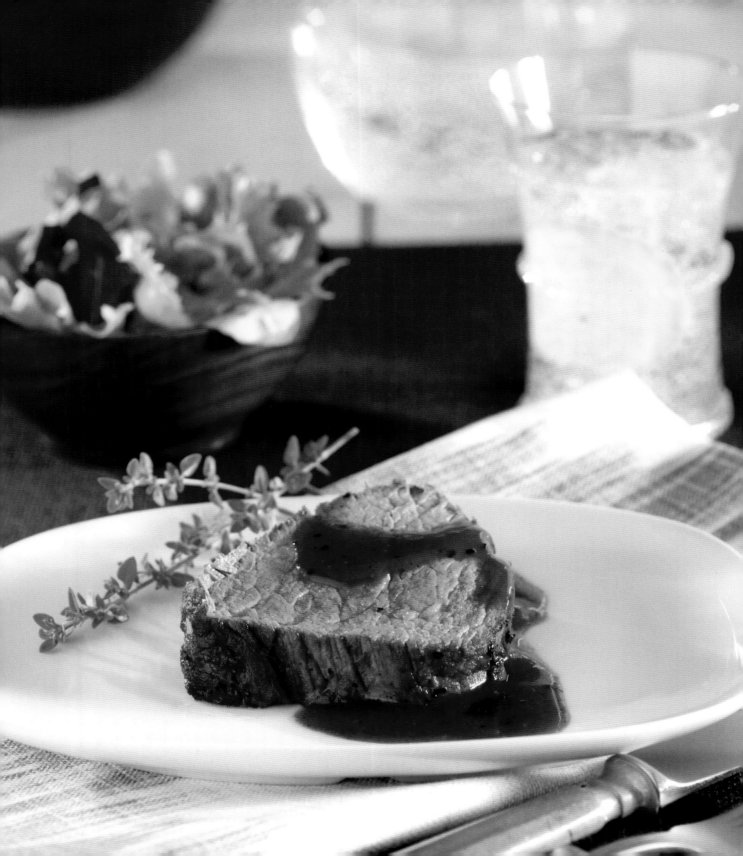

# FLANK STEAK AND ROASTED VEGETABLE SALAD

Makes 4 servings

1½ pounds asparagus spears, trimmed and cut into 2-inch lengths

8 ounces baby carrots (about 2 cups)

2 tablespoons olive oil, divided

1 teaspoon salt, divided

1 teaspoon black pepper, divided

1 pound beef flank steak (1 inch thick)

2 tablespoons plus 1 teaspoon Dijon mustard, divided

1 tablespoon lemon juice

1 tablespoon water

1 teaspoon honey

6 cups mixed salad greens

1. Preheat oven to 400°F. Combine asparagus and carrots, 1 tablespoon oil, ½ teaspoon salt and ¼ teaspoon pepper on baking sheet; toss to coat. Spread vegetables in single layer.

2. Roast 20 minutes or until vegetables are browned and tender, stirring once.

3. Meanwhile, sprinkle steak with ¼ teaspoon salt and ½ teaspoon pepper. Rub both sides of steak with 2 tablespoons mustard. Place steak on rack in small roasting pan.

4. Roast 10 minutes for medium rare or until desired doneness, turning once. Remove steak to cutting board; tent with foil. Let stand 5 minutes before slicing.

5. Combine lemon juice, water, honey, remaining 1 tablespoon oil, 1 teaspoon mustard, ¼ teaspoon salt and ¼ teaspoon pepper in large bowl; mix well. Drizzle 1 tablespoon dressing over vegetables on baking sheet; toss to coat. Add greens to dressing in large bowl; toss to coat.

6. Divide greens among four plates; top with steak and vegetables.

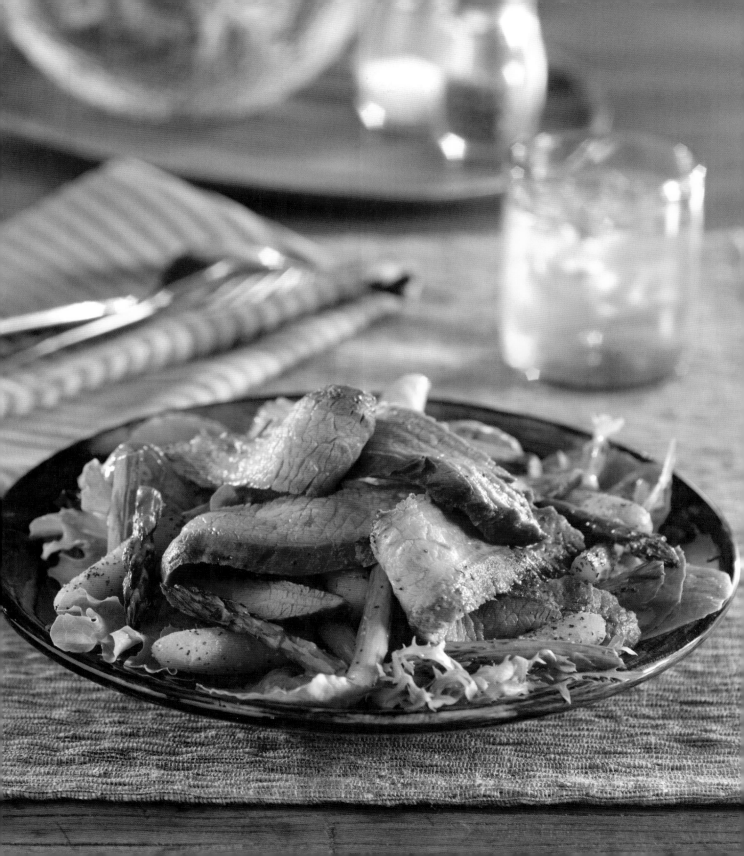

# MARINATED BEEF BROCHETTES

Makes 6 servings

¼ cup finely chopped onion

¼ cup olive oil

3 tablespoons lime juice

1 finely chopped seeded hot finger pepper (about 1 teaspoon)

1 clove garlic, minced

½ teaspoon salt

12 ounces beef tenderloin, cut into 1-inch pieces

1 medium green bell pepper, cut into 1-inch pieces

1 medium red onion, cut into 1-inch pieces

**1.** Combine onion, oil, lime juice, hot pepper, garlic and salt in medium bowl; mix well. Place beef in large resealable food storage bag; pour marinade over beef. Seal bag; turn to coat. Marinate in refrigerator 2 hours or overnight.

**2.** Soak six 8-inch wooden skewers in water 20 minutes before cooking to prevent burning. Oil grid. Prepare grill for direct cooking.

**3.** Remove beef from marinade; discard marinade. Alternately thread beef, bell pepper and onion onto skewers.

**4.** Grill skewers 2 to 3 minutes per side or until desired doneness.

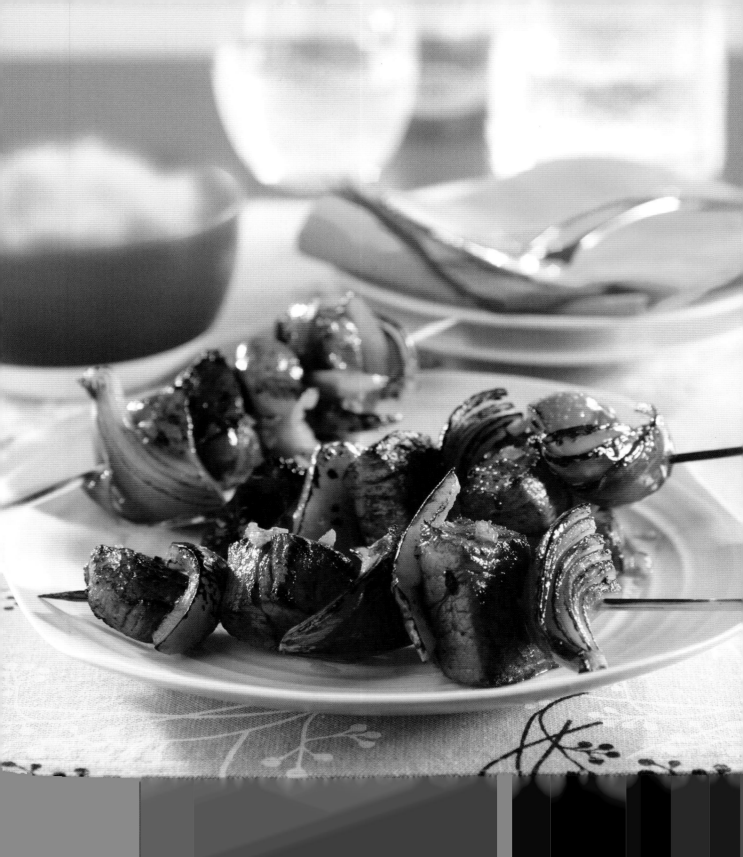

# STEAK DIANE WITH CREMINI MUSHROOMS

### Makes 2 servings

1 tablespoon olive oil, divided

2 beef tenderloin steaks (4 ounces each), ¾ inch thick

¼ teaspoon salt

¼ teaspoon black pepper

⅓ cup sliced shallots or chopped onion

4 ounces cremini mushrooms or mixed wild mushrooms, sliced

1½ tablespoons Paleo Worcestershire Sauce (page 10)

1 tablespoon Dijon mustard

**1.** Heat half of oil in large skillet over medium-high heat. Add steaks; sprinkle with salt and pepper. Cook 3 minutes per side for medium rare or until desired doneness. Remove to plate; tent with foil.

**2.** Add remaining half of oil to skillet; heat over medium heat. Add shallots; cook and stir 2 minutes. Add mushrooms; cook and stir 3 minutes. Add Worcestershire sauce and mustard; cook 1 minute, stirring frequently.

**3.** Return steaks and any accumulated juices to skillet; cook until heated through, turning once. Serve steaks topped with mushroom mixture.

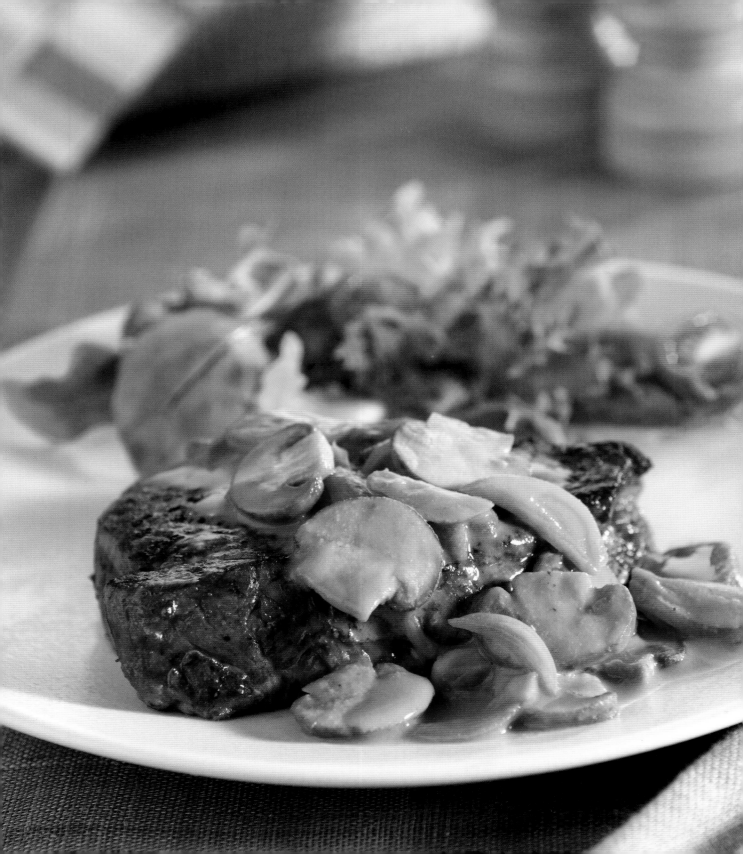

# KOREAN BEEF SHORT RIBS

Makes 4 to 6 servings

¼ cup chopped
   green onions

¼ cup water

¼ cup coconut aminos

1 tablespoon honey

2 teaspoons grated
   fresh ginger

2 teaspoons dark
   sesame oil

2 cloves garlic, minced

½ teaspoon
   black pepper

2½ pounds beef chuck
   flanken-style short
   ribs, ⅜ to ½ inch
   thick*

1 tablespoon sesame
   seeds, toasted

*Flanken-style ribs can be
ordered from your butcher.
They are cross-cut short ribs
sawed through the bones.*

**1.** Combine green onions, water, coconut aminos, honey, ginger, oil, garlic and pepper in small bowl; mix well. Place short ribs in large resealable food storage bag. Pour marinade over ribs. Seal bag; turn to coat. Marinate in refrigerator at least 4 hours or up to 8 hours, turning occasionally.

**2.** Oil grid. Prepare grill for direct cooking. Remove ribs from marinade; reserve marinade.

**3.** Grill ribs, covered, over medium-high heat 5 minutes. Brush with reserved marinade; turn and brush again. Discard remaining marinade. Grill, covered, 5 to 6 minutes for medium or until desired doneness. Sprinkle with sesame seeds.

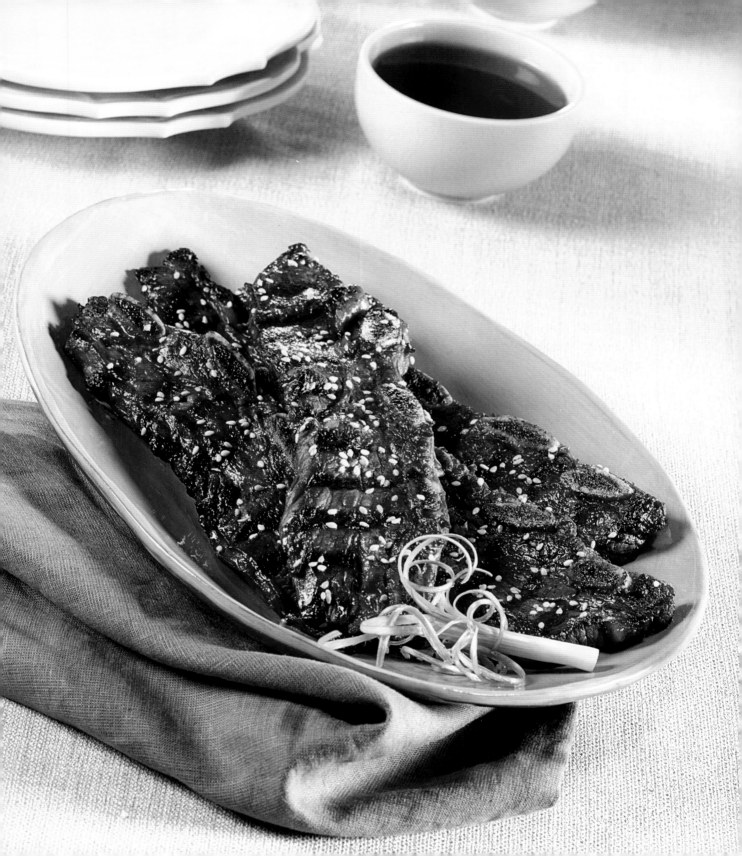

# BEEF AND PEPPER KABOBS

Makes 4 servings

8 ounces sirloin steak

2 tablespoons olive oil

1½ tablespoons red wine vinegar

1½ tablespoons coconut aminos

1 tablespoon Dijon mustard

2 cloves garlic, minced

½ teaspoon salt

¼ teaspoon black pepper

1 tablespoon chicken or vegetable broth

2 medium bell peppers (green, red, yellow or a combination), each cut into 12 pieces

4 large green onions

1. Cut steak into 16 strips, each about ¼ inch thick. Place in large resealable food storage bag.

2. Combine oil, vinegar, coconut aminos, mustard, garlic, salt and black pepper in small bowl; mix well. Pour half of marinade over beef. Seal bag; turn to coat. Marinate in refrigerator 2 to 3 hours, turning occasionally. Reserve remaining marinade.

3. Oil grid. Prepare grill for direct cooking. Stir broth into reserved marinade.

4. Thread bell peppers onto four metal skewers; grill 5 to 7 minutes per side or until tender and beginning to brown. Add green onions to grill; grill 3 to 5 minutes or until well browned on both sides. Brush vegetables lightly with marinade once during grilling. Coarsely chop green onions after grilling.

5. Thread beef strips onto four metal skewers. Grill 2 minutes per side, brushing twice with marinade. Remove beef and bell peppers from skewers; sprinkle with green onions.

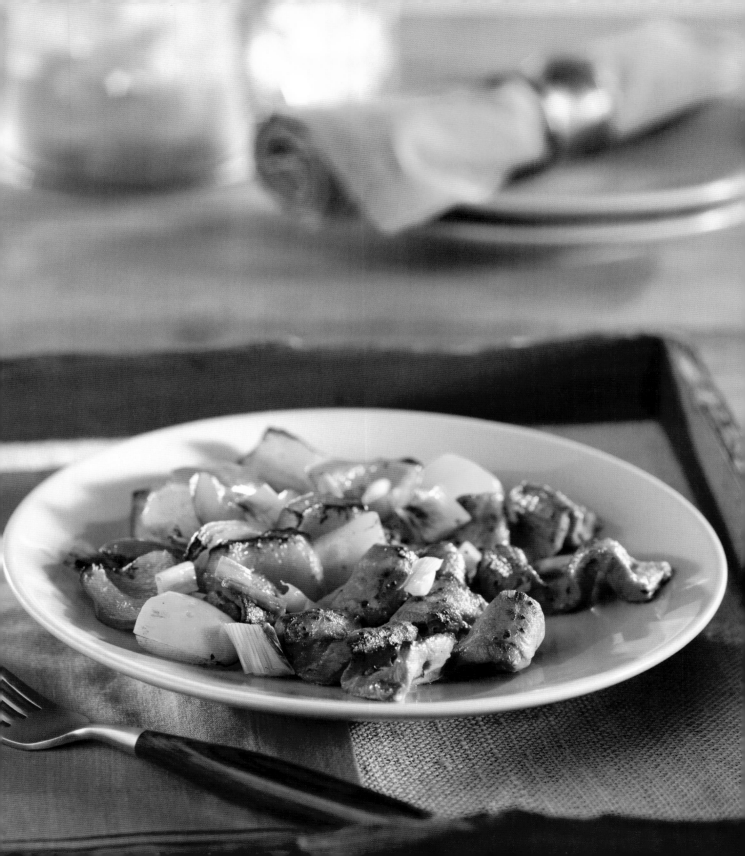

# SESAME-GARLIC FLANK STEAK

Makes 4 servings

1 beef flank steak
  (about 1¼ pounds)

2 tablespoons
  coconut aminos

2 tablespoons Paleo
  Hoisin Sauce
  (page 11)

1 tablespoon dark
  sesame oil

2 cloves garlic, minced

**1.** Score steak lightly with sharp knife in diamond pattern on both sides; place in large resealable food storage bag.

**2.** Combine coconut aminos, hoisin sauce, sesame oil and garlic in small bowl; mix well. Pour marinade over steak. Seal bag; turn to coat. Marinate in refrigerator at least 2 hours or up to 24 hours, turning once.

**3.** Preheat broiler or prepare grill for direct cooking. Line broiler pan or baking sheet with foil. Remove steak from marinade; reserve marinade. Place steak on prepared pan.

**4.** Broil or grill steak 5 to 6 minutes or until browned; turn and brush with reserved marinade. Broil 5 minutes or until 125°F for medium rare or 130° to 135°F for medium or until desired doneness. Discard remaining marinade. Remove steak to cutting board; tent with foil. Let stand 5 minutes before slicing. Cut into thin slices across the grain.

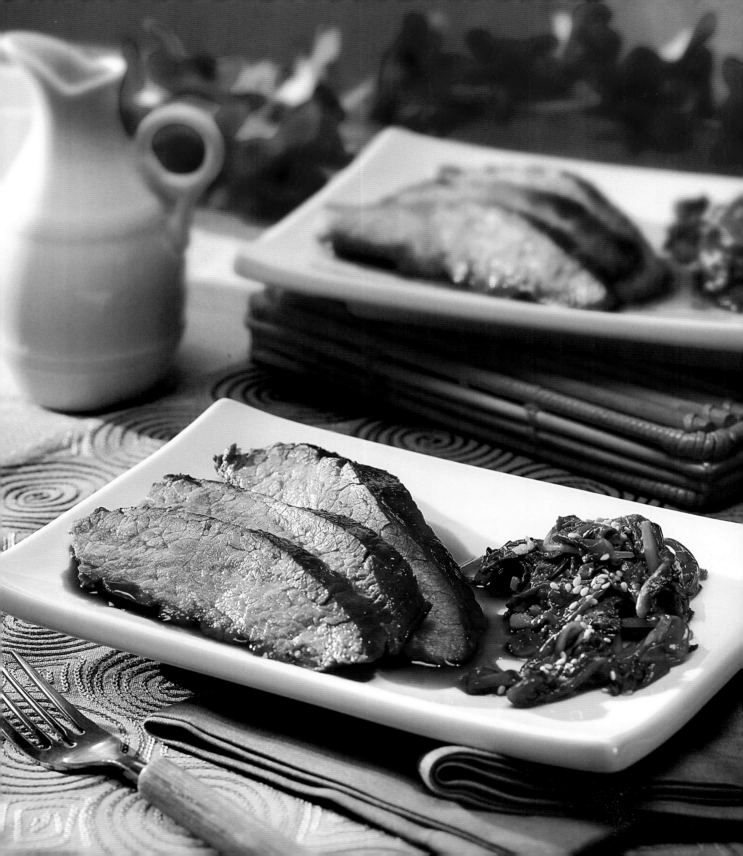

# BEEF POT ROAST

Makes 8 servings

1 tablespoon olive oil

1 boneless beef eye
  of round roast
  (about 2½ pounds),
  trimmed

1 can (about
  14 ounces)
  beef broth

2 cloves garlic

1 teaspoon herbes
  de Provence *or*
  ¼ teaspoon each
  dried rosemary,
  thyme, sage and
  savory

4 small turnips, peeled
  and cut into wedges

10 ounces brussels
  sprouts (about
  10 medium),
  trimmed

8 ounces baby carrots
  (about 2 cups)

4 ounces pearl onions
  (about 1 cup),
  skins removed

**1.** Heat oil in Dutch oven over medium-high heat. Add beef; cook until browned on all sides.

**2.** Add broth, garlic and herbes de Provence to Dutch oven; bring to a boil over high heat. Reduce heat to low; cover and cook 1½ hours.

**3.** Add turnips, brussels sprouts, carrots and onions to Dutch oven; cover and cook over medium heat 25 to 30 minutes or until vegetables are tender. Remove beef and vegetables to serving platter; tent with foil.

**4.** Strain cooking liquid; return to Dutch oven. Bring to a boil over medium-high heat; cook until sauce is reduced and thickened slightly. Serve immediately with pot roast and vegetables.

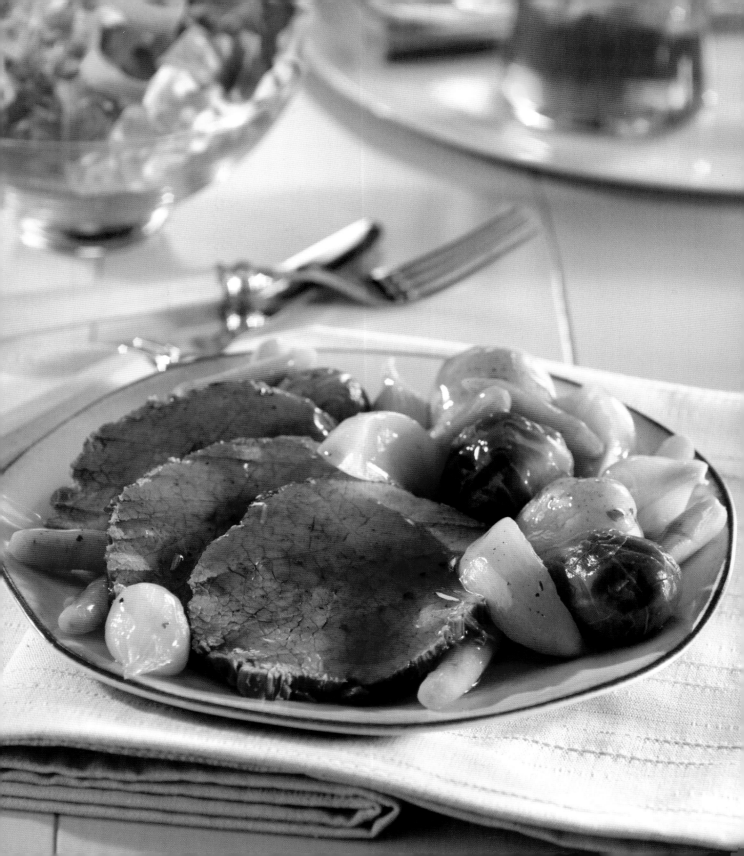

# BEEF TENDERLOIN
# WITH HIGH SPICE RUB

Makes 6 to 8 servings

1 tablespoon
 onion powder

2 teaspoons
 dried thyme

1 teaspoon
 ground cumin

¾ teaspoon
 ground allspice

1 teaspoon
 black pepper

⅛ teaspoon ground
 red pepper

½ teaspoon salt

2 pounds beef
 tenderloin

1 tablespoon olive oil

¼ cup water

**1.** Combine onion powder, thyme, cumin, allspice, black pepper, red pepper and salt in small bowl; mix well. Rub mixture over all sides of beef, pressing firmly for seasonings to adhere. Wrap tightly with plastic wrap; refrigerate 24 hours.

**2.** Preheat oven to 400°F. Line shallow roasting pan or baking sheet with foil.

**3.** Heat oil in large skillet over medium-high heat. Add beef; cook 3 minutes or until well browned. Turn beef; cook 2 minutes or until browned. Remove beef to prepared pan. Add water to skillet; cook 15 seconds, scraping up browned bits from bottom of skillet. Drizzle liquid over beef.

**4.** Roast 25 minutes or until 135°F or for medium rare or until desired doneness. Remove to cutting board; tent with foil. Let stand 10 minutes before slicing.

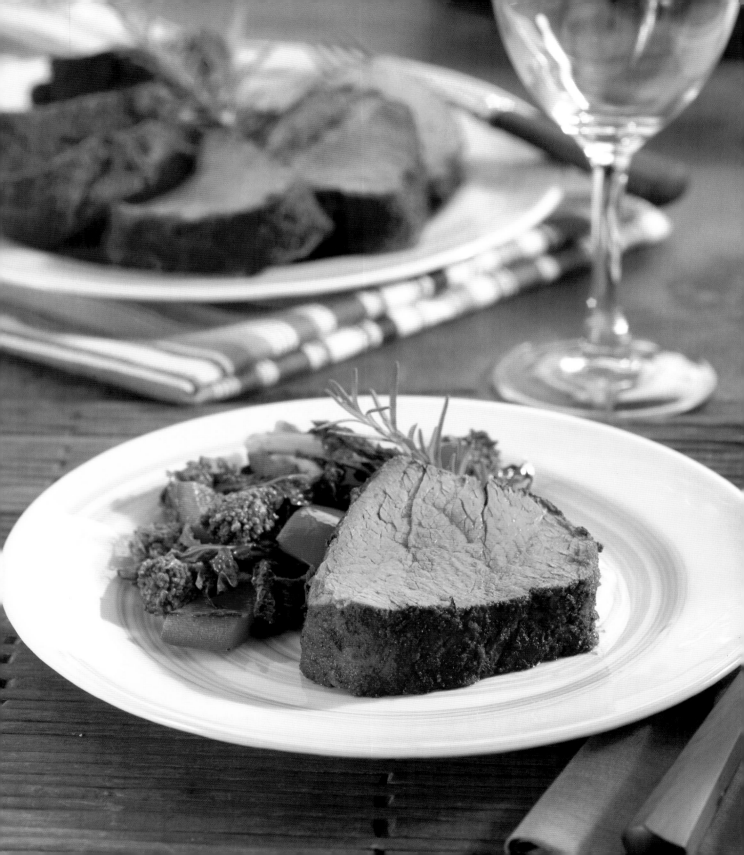

# WARM STEAK SALAD WITH MUSTARD DRESSING

Makes 4 servings

Mustard Dressing
(recipe follows)

1 beef flank steak
(about 1¼ pounds)

Salt and black pepper

4 ounces sugar snap
peas or snow peas

4 cups mixed greens

1 medium red onion,
sliced and separated
into rings

1 pint cherry tomatoes,
halved

**1.** Preheat broiler. Position oven rack about 4 inches from heat source.

**2.** Prepare Mustard Dressing; set aside.

**3.** Place steak on rack of broiler pan. Broil 13 to 18 minutes for medium rare to medium or until desired doneness, turning once. Season with salt and pepper. Remove steak to cutting board; tent with foil. Let stand 5 minutes before slicing.

**4.** Meanwhile, bring lightly salted water to a boil in small saucepan over high heat. Add snap peas; cook 2 minutes. Drain.

**5.** Combine greens, onion, tomatoes and snap peas in medium bowl; toss gently. Divide among four plates.

**6.** Cut steak into thin slices across the grain; arrange over salad. Serve with dressing.

**MUSTARD DRESSING:** Whisk ¾ cup extra virgin olive oil, 3 tablespoons seasoned rice vinegar, 1 tablespoon balsamic vinegar, 1 tablespoon Dijon mustard, ½ teaspoon salt, ¼ teaspoon dried thyme and ⅛ teaspoon black pepper in medium bowl until well blended. Makes about 1 cup.

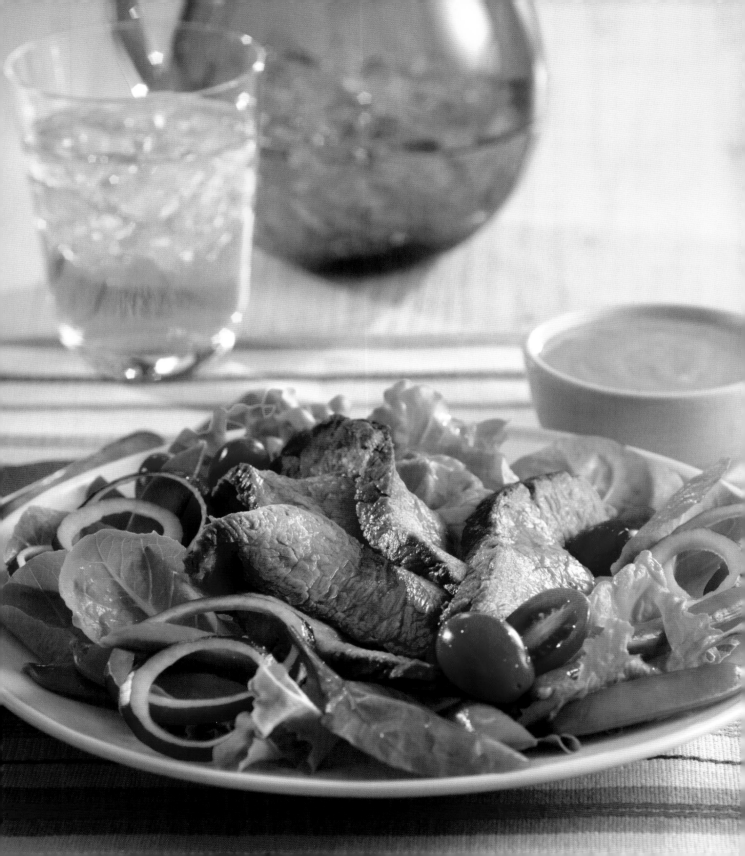

# OLD-FASHIONED BEEF STEW

Makes 6 servings

2 tablespoons olive oil, divided

1½ pounds beef top or bottom round steak, cut into 1-inch pieces

4 cups sliced mushrooms

2 cloves garlic, minced

2 cups baby carrots

2 cups beef broth

2 tablespoons tomato paste

1 teaspoon salt

¾ teaspoon dried thyme

½ teaspoon black pepper

2 bay leaves

2 medium onions, cut into wedges

2 cups frozen cut green beans

2 tablespoons cold water

2 teaspoons arrowroot or tapioca starch

**1.** Heat 1 tablespoon oil in Dutch oven over medium-high heat. Add beef in two batches; cook about 5 minutes or until browned, stirring occasionally. Remove to plate.

**2.** Add remaining 1 tablespoon oil to Dutch oven. Add mushrooms; cook about 8 minutes or until browned, stirring occasionally. Add garlic; cook and stir 30 seconds. Add beef, carrots, broth, tomato paste, salt, thyme, pepper and bay leaves; bring to a boil over medium-high heat. Reduce heat to medium-low; cover and cook 2 hours or until beef is fork-tender. Add onions and green beans during last 30 minutes of cooking.

**3.** Remove and discard bay leaves. Stir water into arrowroot in small bowl until smooth. Slowly stir mixture into stew; cook and stir over low heat 2 to 3 minutes or just until thickened.

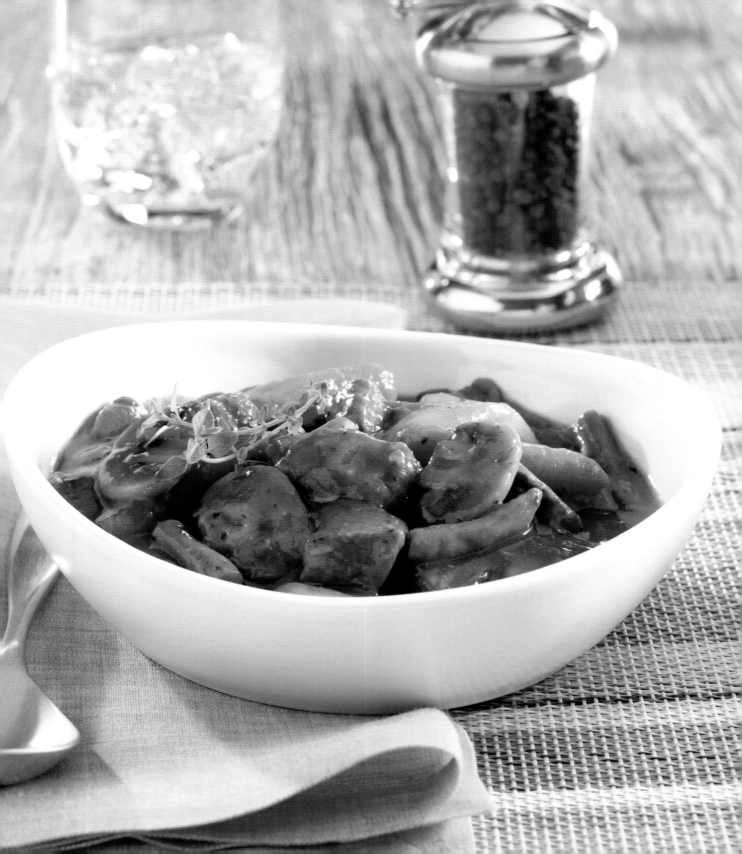

# GRILLED STRIP STEAKS WITH CHIMICHURRI

Makes 4 servings

Chimichurri
(recipe follows)

4 bone-in strip steaks
(8 ounces each),
about 1 inch thick

¾ teaspoon salt

¾ teaspoon
ground cumin

¼ teaspoon
black pepper

**1.** Prepare Chimichurri; set aside.

**2.** Oil grid. Prepare grill for direct cooking. Sprinkle both sides of steaks with salt, cumin and pepper.

**3.** Grill steaks, covered, over medium-high heat 4 to 5 minutes per side for medium rare or until desired doneness. Serve with Chimichurri.

## CHIMICHURRI

Makes about 1 cup

½ cup packed fresh
basil leaves

⅓ cup extra virgin olive oil

¼ cup packed fresh parsley

2 tablespoons packed
fresh cilantro

2 tablespoons lemon juice

1 clove garlic

½ teaspoon salt

½ teaspoon grated
orange peel

¼ teaspoon
ground coriander

⅛ teaspoon black pepper

Combine all ingredients in food processor or blender; process until almost smooth.

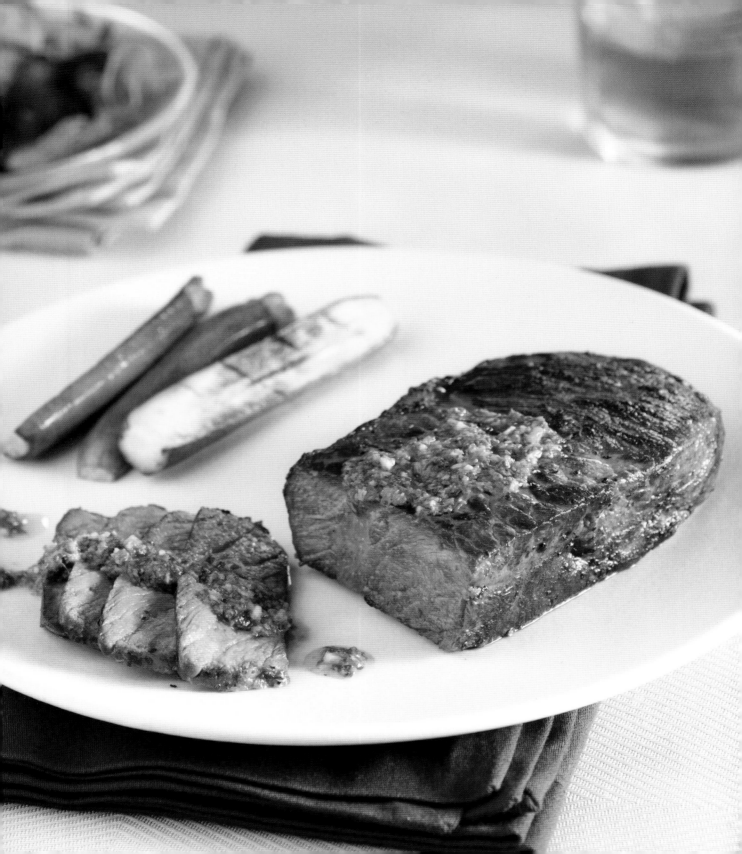

# GINGER BEEF AND CARROT KABOBS

Makes 4 servings

¼ cup coconut aminos

1 tablespoon water

1 tablespoon honey

1 teaspoon olive oil

¼ teaspoon ground ginger

¼ teaspoon ground allspice

⅛ teaspoon ground red pepper

1 clove garlic, minced

12 ounces boneless beef top sirloin steak (1 inch thick), cut into 1-inch pieces

2 medium carrots, cut into 1-inch pieces (1½ cups)

4 green onions, trimmed and cut into 4-inch pieces

1. Combine coconut aminos, water, honey, oil, ginger, allspice, red pepper and garlic in small bowl; mix well. Place beef in large resealable food storage bag. Pour marinade over beef. Seal bag; turn to coat. Marinate in refrigerator 4 to 16 hours, turning occasionally.

2. Meanwhile, bring 1 inch water to a boil in medium saucepan over medium-high heat. Add carrots; cover and cook 5 minutes or until crisp-tender. Drain.

3. Soak four wooden skewers in water 20 minutes to prevent burning. Oil grid. Prepare grill for direct cooking.

4. Remove beef from marinade; discard marinade. Alternately thread beef and carrot pieces onto skewers. Add green onion piece to end of each skewer.

5. Grill skewers over medium heat 11 to 14 minutes or until beef is tender, turning once.

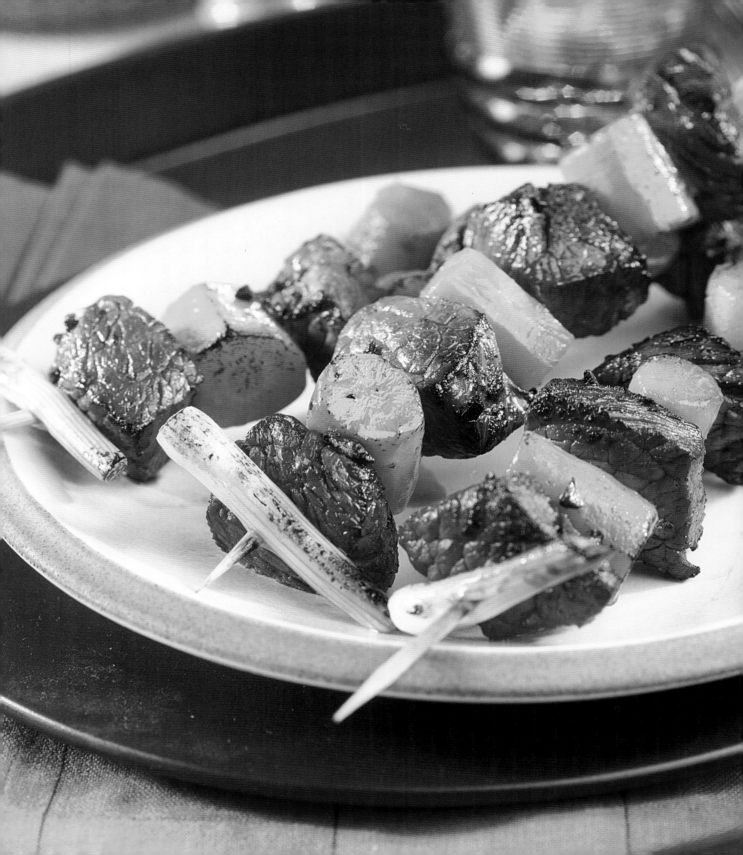

# RIBEYE STEAKS WITH CHILI BUTTER

Makes 4 servings

4 tablespoons (½ stick) butter, softened

1 teaspoon chili powder

½ teaspoon minced garlic

½ teaspoon Dijon mustard

⅛ teaspoon ground red pepper or chipotle chili powder

4 beef rib eye steaks

1 teaspoon black pepper

**1.** Beat butter, chili powder, garlic, mustard and red pepper in medium bowl until smooth.

**2.** Place mixture on sheet of waxed paper. Roll mixture back and forth into 4-inch log using waxed paper. If butter is too soft, refrigerate up to 30 minutes. Wrap with waxed paper; refrigerate at least 1 hour or up to 2 days.

**3.** Oil grid. Prepare grill for direct cooking. Rub black pepper over both sides of steaks.

**4.** Grill steaks, covered, over medium-high heat 8 to 10 minutes or until desired doneness, turning occasionally. Serve with chili butter.

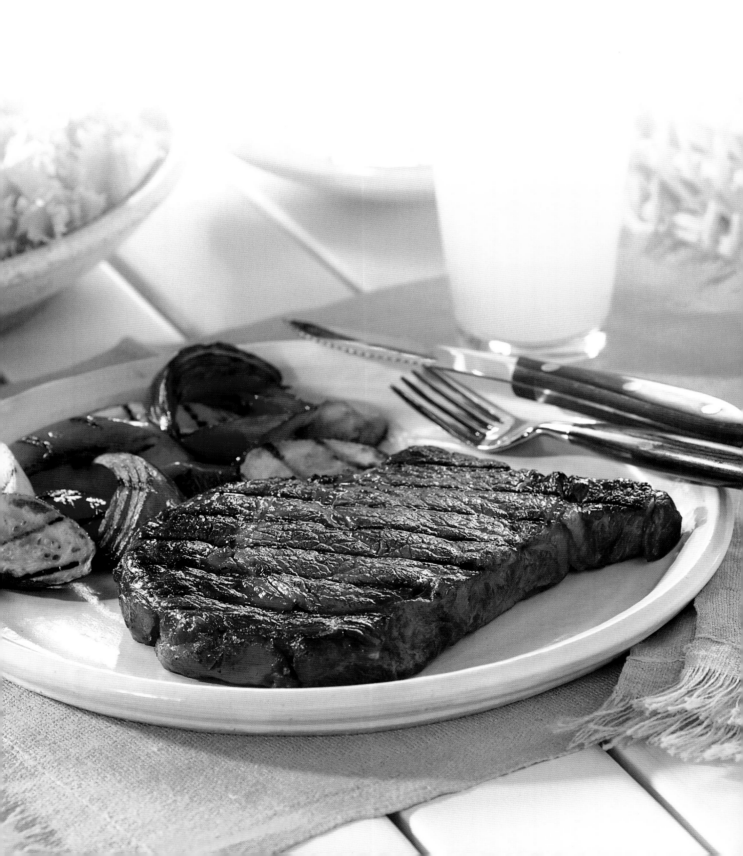

# MUSTARD CRUSTED RIB ROAST

Makes 6 to 8 servings

1 (3-rib) beef rib roast (6 to 7 pounds), trimmed*

3 tablespoons Dijon mustard

1½ tablespoons chopped fresh tarragon *or* 1½ teaspoons dried tarragon

3 cloves garlic, minced

½ teaspoon salt

¼ teaspoon black pepper

¼ cup dry red wine

⅓ cup finely chopped shallots (about 2 shallots)

1 cup beef broth

*Ask butcher to remove chine bone for easier carving. Trim fat to ¼-inch thickness.*

1. Preheat oven to 450°F. Place beef, bone side down, in shallow roasting pan. Combine mustard, tarragon, garlic, salt and pepper in small bowl; mix well. Spread mixture over top and sides of beef. Roast 10 minutes.

2. *Reduce oven temperature to 350°F.* Roast 2½ to 3 hours until 145°F for medium or until desired doneness. Remove beef to cutting board; tent with foil. Let stand 10 to 15 minutes before carving. (Internal temperature will continue to rise 5° to 10°F during stand time.)

3. Meanwhile, measure 1 tablespoon drippings from roasting pan; place in medium saucepan. Discard remaining drippings.

4. Add wine to roasting pan; place over two burners. Cook and stir over medium heat 2 minutes or until slightly thickened, scraping up browned bits from bottom of pan.

5. Add shallots to reserved drippings in saucepan; cook and stir over medium heat 4 minutes or until softened. Add broth and wine mixture; cook about 8 minutes or until sauce is reduced slightly, stirring occasionally. Pour through fine-mesh strainer before serving.

6. Cut roast into ½-inch-thick slices. Serve with sauce.

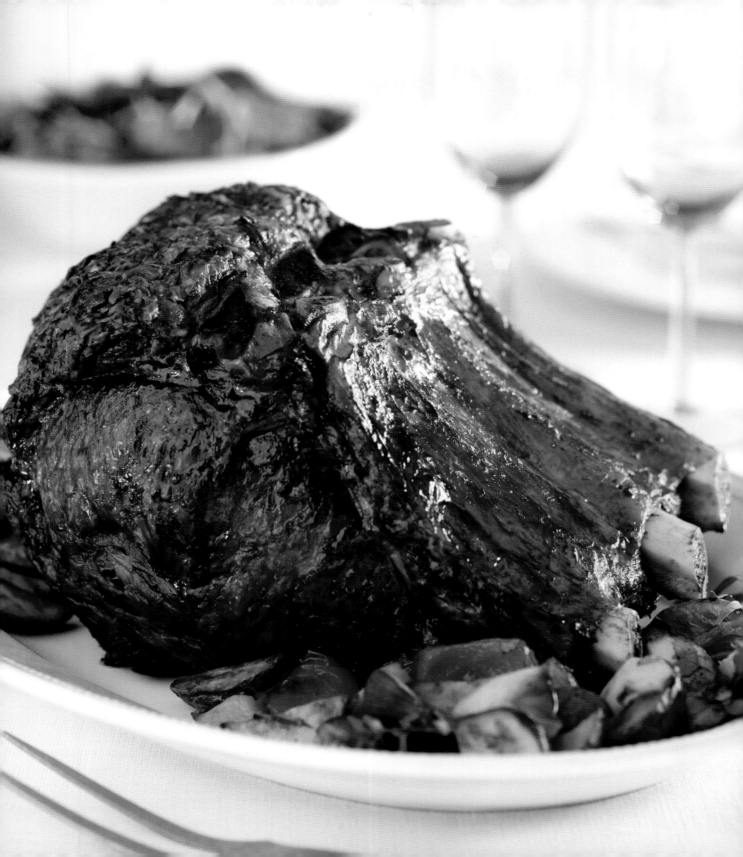

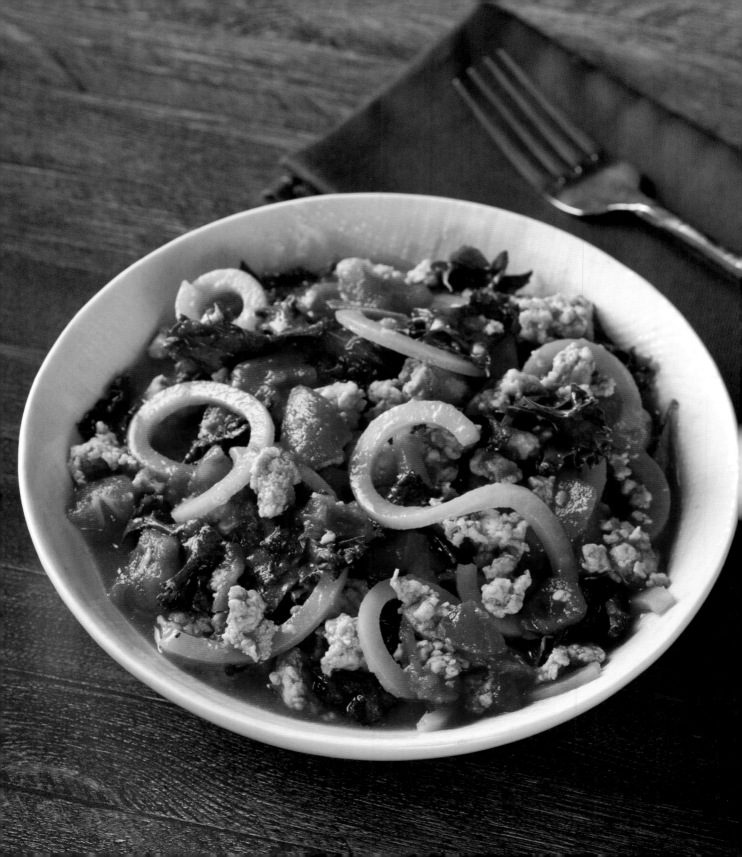

# PORK & LAMB

## SAUSAGE, SQUASH AND KALE STEW

Makes 4 servings

1 small butternut squash, peeled

1 tablespoon olive oil

12 ounces hot or mild Italian pork or turkey sausage

6 cups coarsely chopped stemmed kale or Swiss chard (about 4 ounces)

1 can (about 14 ounces) diced tomatoes

½ cup water

¼ teaspoon black pepper

**1.** Use spiralizer to spiral squash with thick ribbon blade; cut into desired lengths.*

**2.** Heat oil in large saucepan over medium heat. Remove sausage from casings; crumble into saucepan. Cook over medium heat until browned, stirring to break up meat.

**3.** Stir in kale, tomatoes and water; cover and cook over medium-low heat 8 minutes. Stir in squash and pepper; cover and cook 5 minutes or until squash is tender.

*If you don't have a spiralizer, cut squash into ½-inch pieces. Add squash to saucepan with kale at the beginning of step 3.*

# CUBAN GARLIC AND LIME PORK CHOPS

Makes 4 servings

2 tablespoons olive oil

2 tablespoons lime juice

2 tablespoons orange juice

2 teaspoons minced garlic

½ teaspoon salt, divided

½ teaspoon red pepper flakes

4 boneless pork top loin chops (about 6 ounces each), ¾ inch thick

2 small seedless oranges, peeled and chopped

1 medium cucumber, peeled, seeded and chopped

2 tablespoons chopped onion

2 tablespoons chopped fresh cilantro

**1.** Combine oil, lime juice, orange juice, garlic, ¼ teaspoon salt and red pepper flakes in small bowl; mix well. Place pork in large resealable food storage bag. Pour marinade over pork. Seal bag; turn to coat. Marinate in refrigerator up to 24 hours, turning occasionally.

**2.** Combine oranges, cucumber, onion and cilantro in medium bowl; toss gently. Cover and refrigerate salsa at least 1 hour or overnight. Add remaining ¼ teaspoon salt just before serving.

**3.** Prepare grill for direct cooking or preheat broiler. Remove pork from marinade; discard marinade.

**4.** Grill or broil pork 6 to 8 minutes per side or until barely pink in center. Serve with salsa.

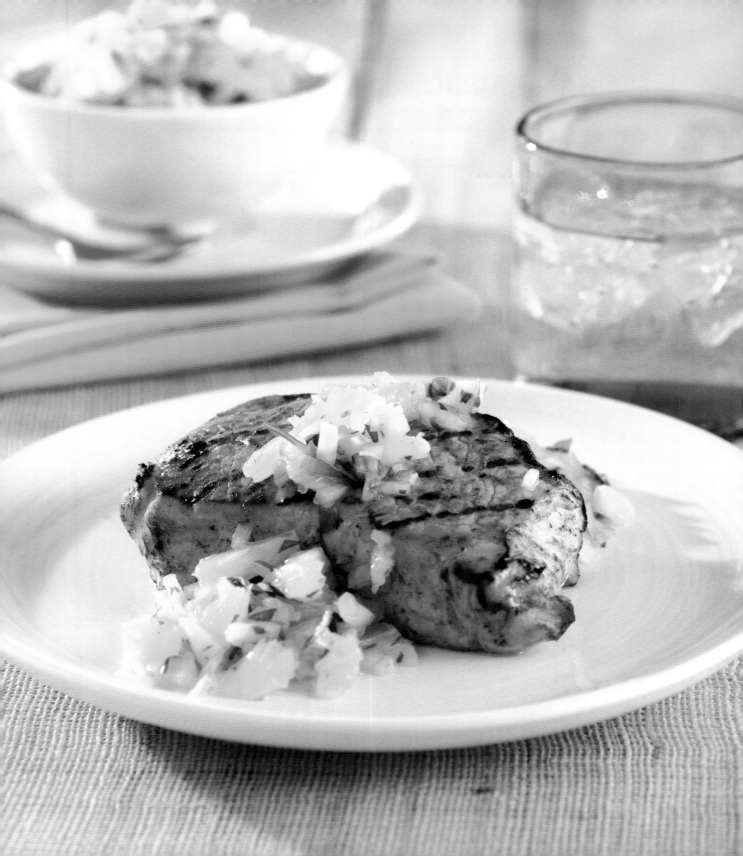

# SWEET GINGERED SPARERIBS

Makes 4 to 6 servings

½ cup coconut aminos

⅓ cup honey

¼ cup dry sherry

1 clove garlic, minced

½ teaspoon ground ginger

4 pounds pork spareribs, cut into 1- or 2-rib pieces

**1.** Preheat oven to 350°F. Line baking sheet with foil.

**2.** Combine coconut aminos, honey, sherry, garlic and ginger in small bowl; mix well.

**3.** Arrange ribs on prepared baking sheet, meat side down. Brush honey mixture generously over ribs. Cover loosely with foil.

**4.** Bake 1 hour. Turn ribs; brush with additional honey mixture. Bake, uncovered, 30 minutes or until ribs are tender, brushing occasionally with remaining honey mixture.

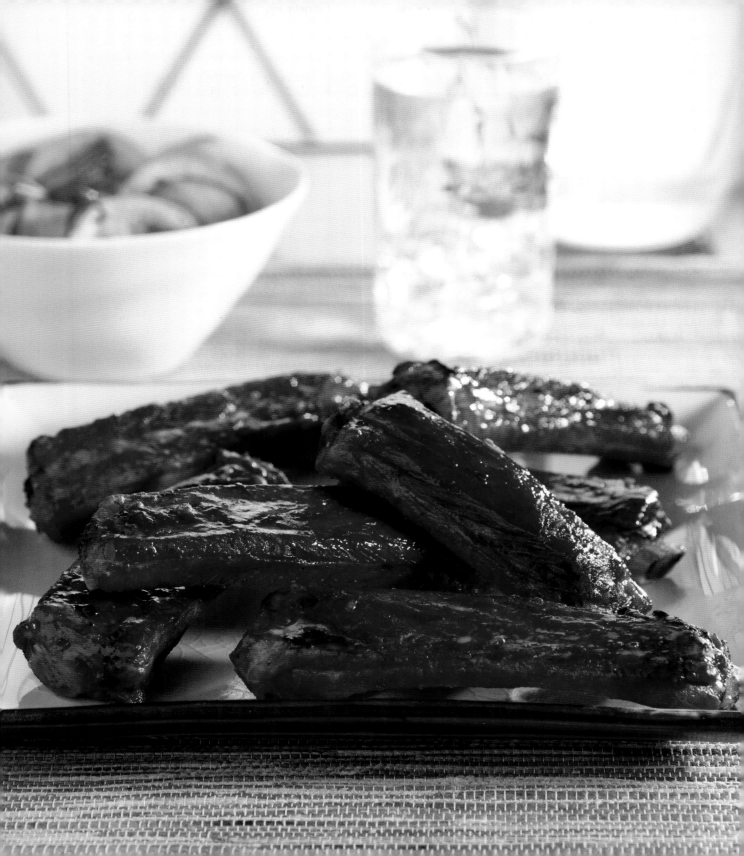

# HERBED LAMB CHOPS

Makes 4 servings

⅓ cup olive oil

⅓ cup red wine vinegar

2 tablespoons coconut aminos

1 tablespoon lemon juice

3 cloves garlic, minced

1 teaspoon salt

1 teaspoon chopped fresh oregano *or* ¼ teaspoon dried oregano

1 teaspoon dried rosemary

1 teaspoon ground mustard

½ teaspoon white pepper

8 lamb loin chops, (about 4 ounces each), 1 inch thick

**1.** Combine oil, vinegar, coconut aminos, lemon juice, garlic, salt, oregano, rosemary, mustard and pepper in large resealable food storage bag. Reserve ½ cup marinade in small bowl; set aside. Add lamb to remaining marinade. Seal bag; turn to coat. Marinate in refrigerator at least 1 hour.

**2.** Prepare grill for direct cooking. Remove lamb from marinade; discard marinade.

**3.** Grill lamb over medium-high heat 4 to 5 minutes per side or until desired doneness, basting frequently with reserved ½ cup marinade. Do not baste during last 5 minutes of cooking. Discard any remaining marinade.

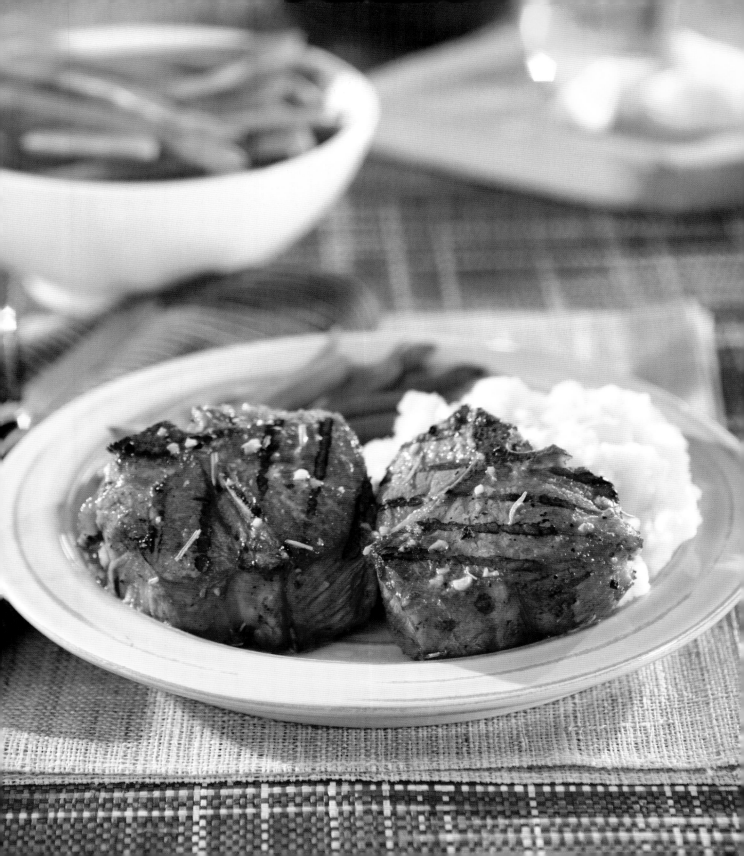

# ROSEMARY PORK TENDERLOIN AND VEGETABLES

### Makes 6 servings

1½ tablespoons olive oil, divided

¼ cup chicken broth

3 large parsnips, peeled and cut diagonally into ½-inch slices

2 cups baby carrots

1 red bell pepper, cut into ¾-inch pieces

1 medium sweet or yellow onion, cut into wedges

2 small pork tenderloins (12 ounces each)

2 tablespoons Dijon mustard

2 teaspoons dried rosemary

¾ teaspoon salt

½ teaspoon black pepper

**1.** Preheat oven to 400°F. Brush shallow roasting pan or baking sheet with ½ tablespoon oil.

**2.** Combine broth and remaining 1 tablespoon oil in small bowl; mix well. Combine parsnips, carrots and 3 tablespoons broth mixture in prepared pan; toss to coat. Spread vegetables in single layer; roast 10 minutes.

**3.** Add bell pepper, onion and remaining broth mixture to pan; toss to coat. Push vegetables to edges of pan. Place pork in center of pan; spread with mustard. Sprinkle pork and vegetables with rosemary, salt and black pepper.

**4.** Roast 25 to 30 minutes or until vegetables are tender and pork is 145°F. Remove pork to cutting board; tent with foil. Let stand 10 minutes before slicing.

**5.** Cut pork into ½-inch slices; serve with vegetables and any juices from pan.

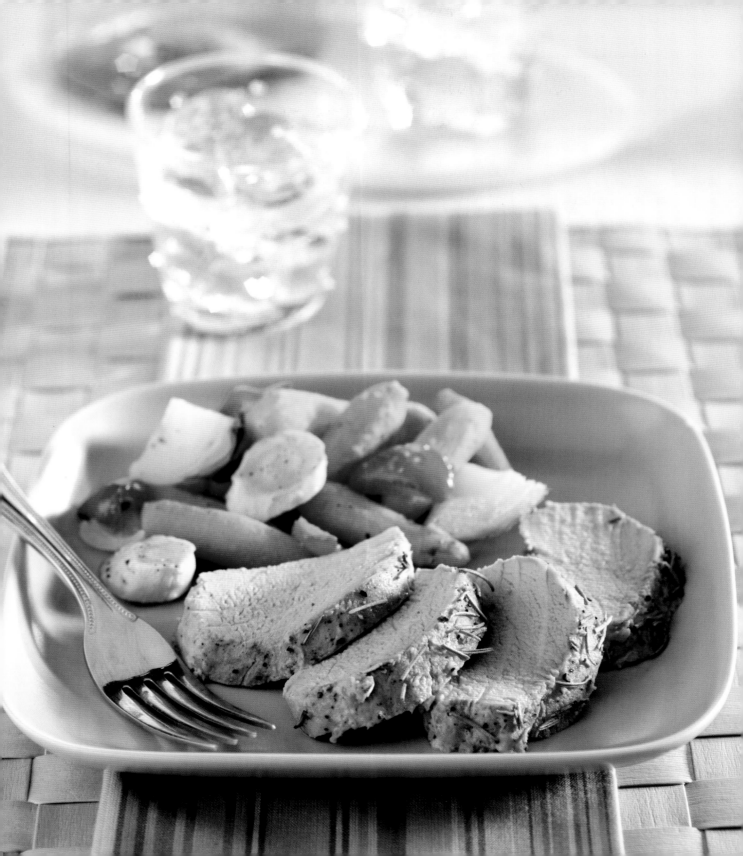

# HONEY GINGER RIBS

Makes about 4 servings

½ cup Paleo Hoisin
   Sauce (page 11)

3 tablespoons
   dry sherry

2 tablespoons honey

2 tablespoons
   coconut aminos

1 tablespoon
   cider vinegar

1 teaspoon minced
   fresh ginger

2 cloves garlic, minced

¼ teaspoon Chinese
   five-spice powder

3 pounds pork
   baby back ribs

Sesame seeds
   (optional)

**1.** Combine hoisin sauce, sherry, honey, coconut aminos, vinegar, ginger, garlic and five-spice powder in small bowl; mix well. Reserve ⅓ cup marinade; set aside.

**2.** Cut rack of ribs in half or thirds to fit in large resealable food storag bag. Pour marinade over ribs; seal bag and turn to coat. Marinate in refrigerator 4 hours or overnight, turning occasionally.

**3.** Preheat oven to 300°F. Line baking sheet with foil. Remove ribs from marinade; discard marinade. Place ribs on prepared baking sheet; cover with foil.

**4.** Bake 1 hour. Remove foil; drain off excess liquid. Bake, uncovered, 1 hour or until ribs are tender. *Turn oven to broil.*

**5.** Brush ribs with reserved marinade. Broil about 3 minutes or until ribs begin to char. Sprinkle with sesame seeds, if desired.

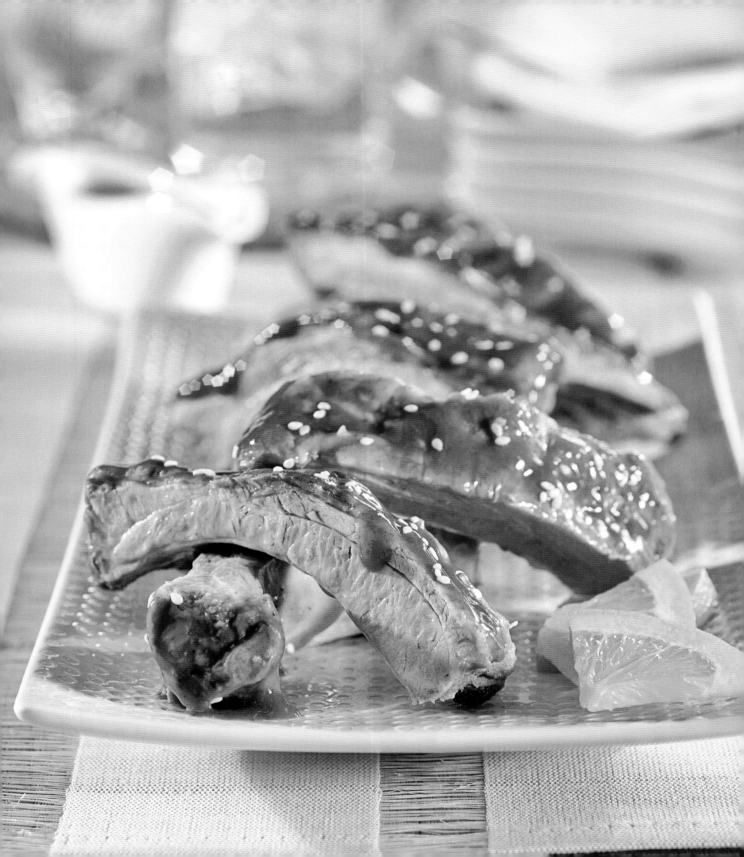

# ZESTY SKILLET PORK CHOPS

Makes 4 servings

1 teaspoon
    chili powder

½ teaspoon salt,
    divided

4 boneless pork chops
    (about 6 ounces
    each)

2 cups diced tomatoes

1 cup chopped
    green, red or
    yellow bell pepper

¾ cup thinly
    sliced celery

½ cup chopped onion

1 teaspoon
    dried thyme

1 tablespoon hot
    pepper sauce

1 tablespoon olive oil

2 tablespoons
    finely chopped
    fresh parsley

**1.** Rub chili powder and ¼ teaspoon salt over one side of pork chops.

**2.** Combine tomatoes, bell pepper, celery, onion, thyme and hot pepper sauce in medium bowl; mix well.

**3.** Heat oil in large skillet over medium-high heat. Add pork, seasoned side down; cook 1 minute. Turn pork and top with tomato mixture; bring to a boil. Reduce heat to low; cover and cook 25 minutes or until pork is tender and sauce has thickened.

**4.** Remove pork to plate; tent with foil. Bring sauce to a boil over high heat; cook 2 minutes or until liquid has almost evaporated. Remove from heat; stir in parsley and remaining ¼ teaspoon salt. Serve over pork.

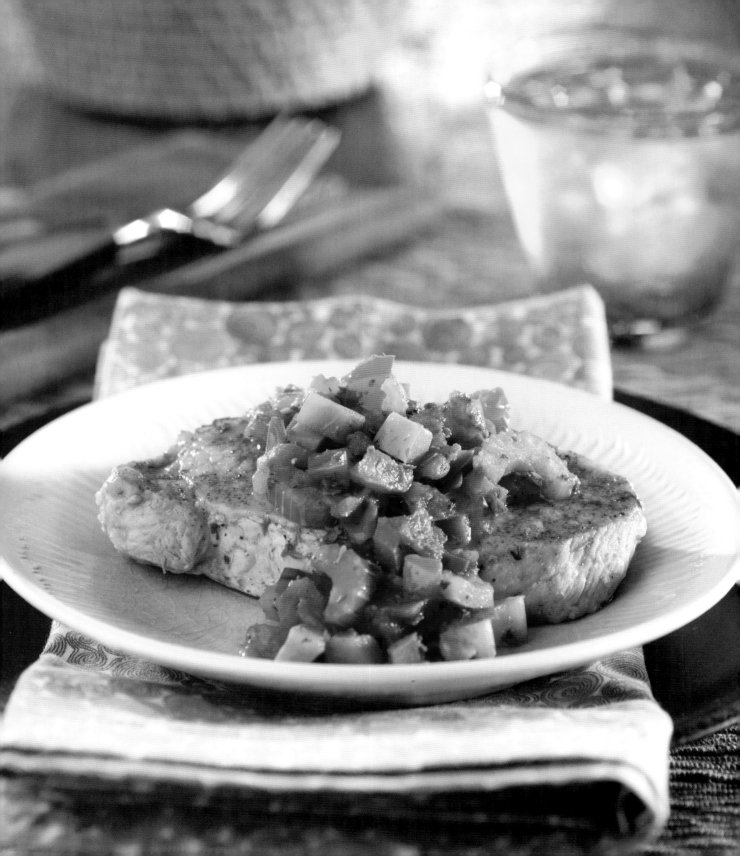

# SAGE-ROASTED PORK WITH RUTABAGA

Makes 4 to 6 servings

1 bunch fresh sage

4 cloves garlic, minced (2 tablespoons)

1½ teaspoons coarse salt, divided

1 teaspoon coarsely ground black pepper, divided

5 tablespoons extra virgin olive oil, divided

1 boneless pork loin roast (2 to 2½ pounds)

2 medium or 1 large rutabaga (1 to 1½ pounds)

4 carrots, cut into 1½-inch pieces

**1.** Chop enough sage to measure 2 tablespoons; reserve remaining sage. Mash chopped sage, garlic, ½ teaspoon salt and ½ teaspoon pepper in small bowl to form paste. Stir in 2 tablepoons oil.

**2.** Score fatty side of pork roast with sharp knife, making cuts about ¼ inch deep. Rub herb paste into cuts and over all sides of pork. Place pork on large plate; cover and refrigerate 1 to 2 hours.

**3.** Preheat oven to 400°F. Cut rutabaga into halves or quarters; peel and cut into 1½-inch pieces. Combine rutabaga and carrots in large bowl. Add remaining 3 tablespoons oil, remaining 1 teaspoon salt and ½ teaspoon pepper; toss to coat.

**4.** Arrange vegetables in single layer in large baking dish or roasting pan. Place pork on top of vegetables, scraping any remaining herb paste from plate into pan. Tuck 3 sprigs of remaining sage into vegetables.

**5.** Roast 15 minutes. *Reduce oven temperature to 325°F.* Roast 45 minutes to 1 hour and 15 minutes or until pork is 145°F and barely pink in center, stirring vegetables once or twice during cooking. Remove pork to cutting board; tent with foil. Let stand 10 minutes before slicing.

**TIP:** Rutabagas can be difficult to cut—they are a tough vegetable and slippery on the outside because they are waxed. Cutting them into large pieces (halves or quarters) before peeling and chopping) makes them easier to manage.

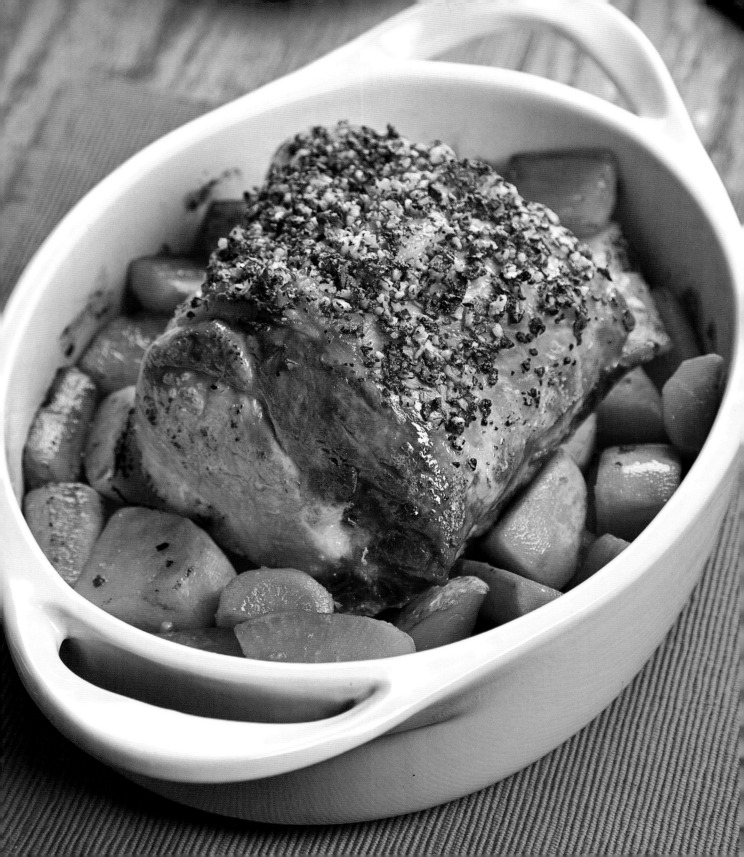

# ROSEMARY-GARLIC LAMB CHOPS

## Makes 4 servings

2 tablespoons olive oil

2 tablespoons finely chopped fresh rosemary leaves

6 cloves garlic, minced

1 teaspoon salt

½ teaspoon ground black pepper

12 small lamb rib chops, bone-in and frenched*

*The term frenched means that the fat and meat have been cut away from the end of the bone protruding from the chop. Ask the butcher to do this for you if frenched chops are not available already cut. You can also purchase a frenched rack of lamb and cut it into individual chops.

**1.** Combine oil, rosemary, garlic, salt and pepper in small bowl; mix well.

**2.** Rub mixture over both sides of lamb chops; wrap in single layer with foil. Marinate in refrigerator 30 minutes to 3 hours.

**3.** Oil grid. Prepare grill for direct cooking or preheat broiler.

**4.** Grill lamb over medium-high heat 2 to 5 minutes per side or until medium rare (145°F). Lamb should feel slightly firm when pressed. (To check doneness, cut small slit in meat near bone; lamb should be rosy pink.)

**VARIATION:** Add 2 teaspoons Dijon mustard to the marinade.

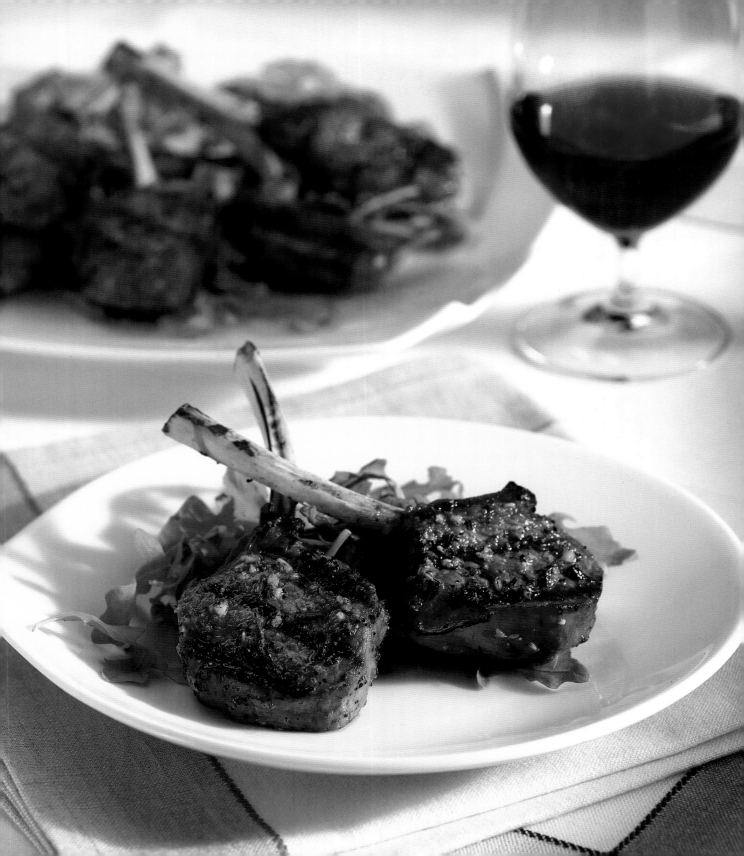

# GRILLED PORK TENDERLOIN WITH APPLE SALSA

Makes 4 servings

1 tablespoon
   chili powder

½ teaspoon
   garlic powder

¾ teaspoon salt,
   divided

1 pound pork
   tenderloin

2 Granny Smith apples,
   peeled, cored and
   finely chopped

1 can (4 ounces) diced
   mild green chiles

¼ cup lemon juice

3 tablespoons
   finely chopped
   fresh cilantro

1 clove garlic, minced

1 teaspoon
   dried oregano

**1.** Oil grid. Prepare grill for direct cooking.

**2.** Combine chili powder, garlic powder and ¼ teaspoon salt in small bowl; mix well. Rub mixture over all sides of pork.

**3.** Grill pork over medium-high heat 30 minutes or until 145°F, turning occasionally. Remove pork to cutting board; tent with foil. Let stand 10 minutes before slicing.

**4.** Meanwhile, combine apples, chiles, lemon juice, cilantro, garlic, oregano and remaining ½ teaspoon salt in medium bowl; mix well.

**5.** Slice pork; serve with salsa. Garnish, if desired.

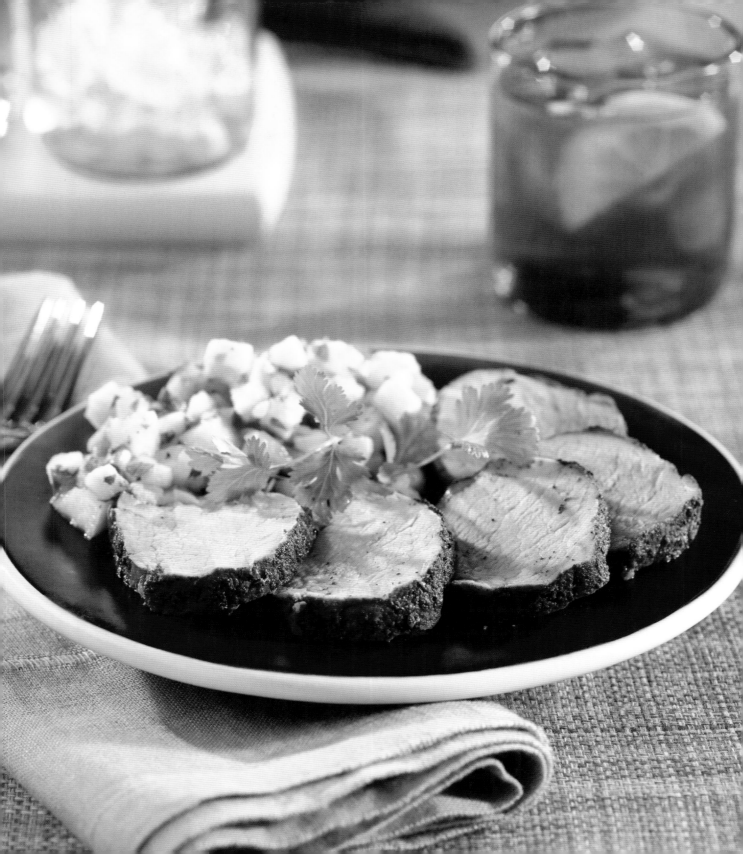

# PORK CURRY OVER CAULIFLOWER COUSCOUS

Makes 6 servings

3 tablespoons olive oil, divided

2 tablespoons mild curry powder

2 teaspoons minced garlic

1½ pounds boneless pork (shoulder, loin or chops), cubed

1 red or green bell pepper, diced

1 tablespoon cider vinegar

½ teaspoon salt

2 cups water

1 large head cauliflower

**1.** Heat 2 tablespoons oil in large saucepan over medium heat. Add curry powder and garlic; cook and stir 1 to 2 minutes or until garlic is golden.

**2.** Add pork; cook and stir 5 to 7 minutes or until barely pink in center. Add bell pepper and vinegar; cook and stir 3 minutes or until bell pepper is soft. Sprinkle with salt.

**3.** Add water; bring to a boil. Reduce heat to low; cook 30 to 45 minutes or until liquid is reduced and pork is tender, stirring occasionally and adding additional water as needed.

**4.** Meanwhile, trim and core cauliflower; cut into 3- to 4-inch pieces. Place in food processor; pulse until cauliflower is in small uniform pieces about the size of cooked couscous.

**5.** Heat remaining 1 tablespoon oil in large skillet over medium heat. Add cauliflower; cook and stir 5 minutes or until crisp-tender. Serve pork curry over cauliflower.

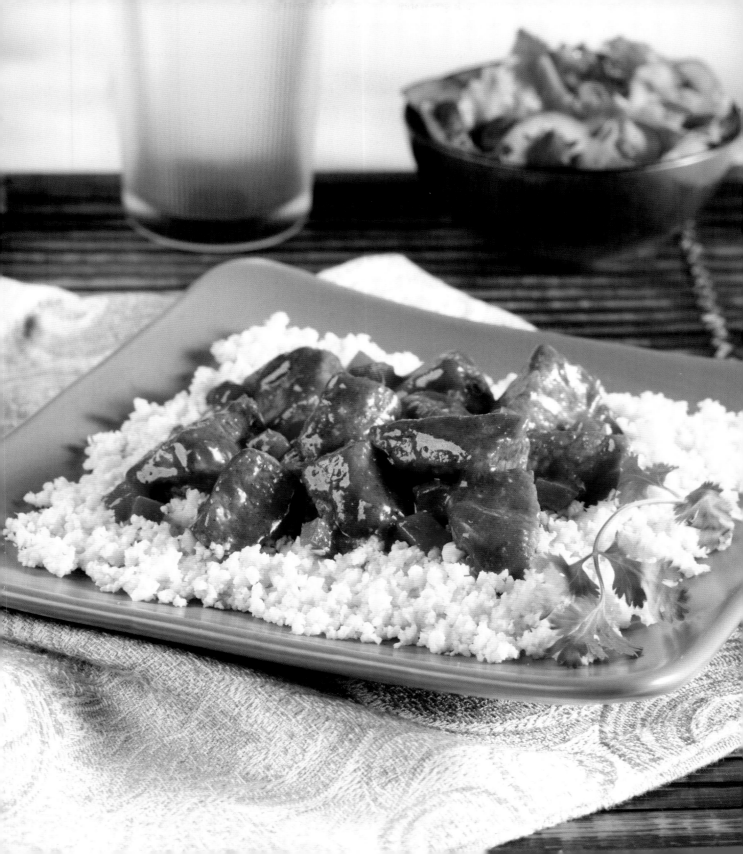

# HERB-ROASTED DIJON LAMB WITH VEGETABLES

Makes 8 to 10 servings

20 cloves garlic, peeled (about 2 medium heads)

¼ cup Dijon mustard

2 tablespoons water

2 tablespoons fresh rosemary leaves

1 tablespoon fresh thyme

1¼ teaspoons salt, divided

1 teaspoon black pepper

4½ pounds boneless leg of lamb, trimmed

1 pound parsnips, cut diagonally into ½-inch pieces

1 pound carrots, cut diagonally into ½-inch pieces

2 large onions, cut into ½-inch wedges

3 tablespoons extra virgin olive oil, divided

**1.** Combine garlic, mustard, water, rosemary, thyme, ¾ teaspoon salt and pepper in food processor; process until smooth. Place lamb in large bowl; spoon garlic mixture over top and sides of lamb. Cover and marinate in refrigerator at least 8 hours.

**2.** Preheat oven to 500°F. Line broiler pan with foil; top with broiler rack. Combine parsnips, carrots, onions and 2 tablespoons oil in large bowl; toss to coat. Spread vegetables on broiler rack; top with lamb.

**3.** Roast 15 minutes. *Reduce oven temperature to 325°F.* Roast 1 hour and 20 minutes until 145°F for medium or until desired doneness. Remove lamb to cutting board; tent with foil. Let stand 10 minutes before slicing. Continue roasting vegetables 10 minutes.

**4.** Transfer vegetables to large bowl. Add remaining 1 tablespoon oil and ½ teaspoon salt; toss to coat. Slice lamb; serve with vegetables.

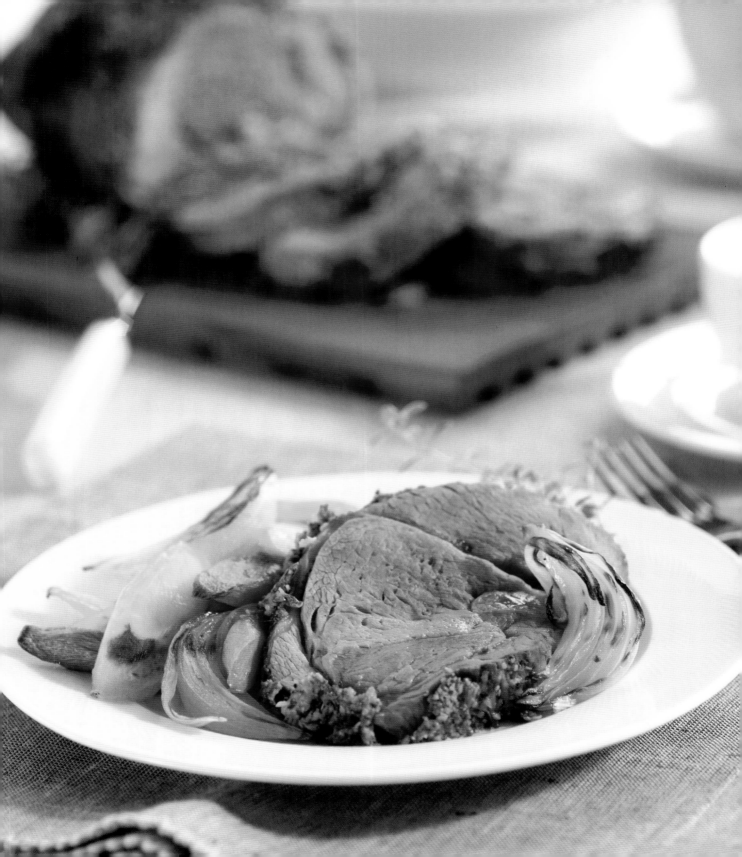

# PORK CHOPS WITH BELL PEPPERS AND SWEET POTATO

Makes 4 servings

4 pork loin chops
  (4 to 6 ounces each),
  about ½ inch thick

1 teaspoon lemon-
  pepper seasoning

1 tablespoon olive oil

½ cup chicken broth

1 tablespoon lemon
  juice

1 teaspoon dried
  fines herbes

¾ teaspoon salt

1¼ cups red and/or
  yellow bell
  pepper strips

1 medium sweet
  potato, peeled,
  quartered and sliced

1 medium onion, sliced

**1.** Rub both sides of pork with lemon-pepper seasoning. Heat oil in large skillet over medium-high heat. Add pork; cook 2 to 3 minutes per side or until browned.

**2.** Combine broth, lemon juice, fines herbes and salt in small bowl; mix well. Pour over pork. Reduce heat to medium-low; cover and cook 5 minutes.

**3.** Add bell pepper, sweet potato and onion to skillet; return to a boil. Reduce heat to low; cover and cook 10 to 15 minutes or until pork is barely pink in center and vegetables are crisp-tender. Remove pork and vegetables to platter; tent with foil.

**4.** Bring remaining liquid in skillet to a boil over high heat. Reduce heat to medium; cook 6 to 8 minutes or until sauce is slightly thickened, stirring occasionally. Pour over pork and vegetables.

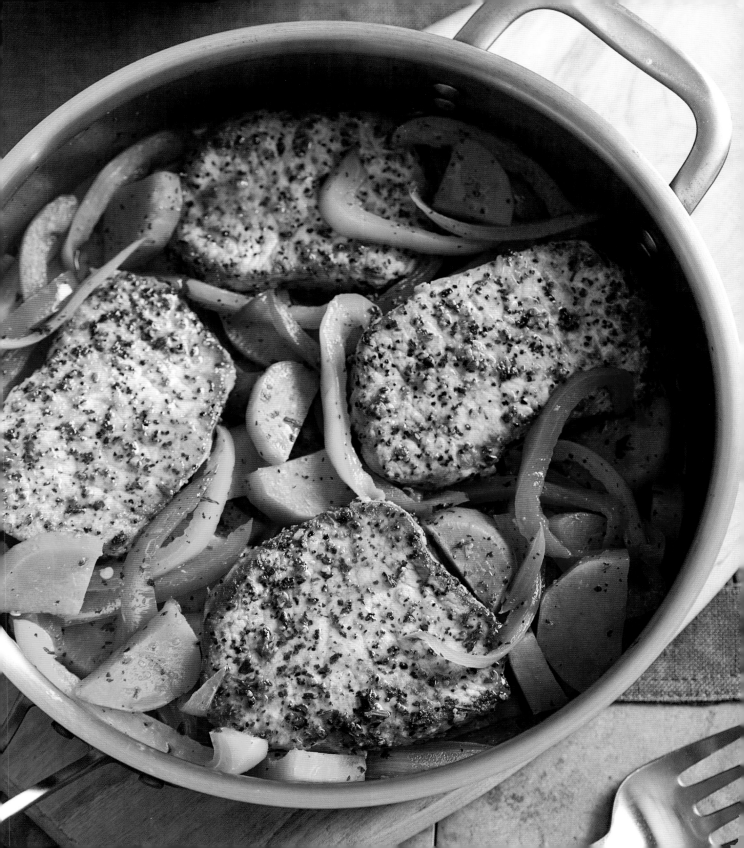

# MOROCCAN-STYLE LAMB CHOPS

Makes 4 servings

1 tablespoon olive oil

1 teaspoon
   ground cumin

1 teaspoon
   ground coriander

¾ teaspoon salt

⅛ teaspoon
   ground cinnamon

⅛ teaspoon ground
   red pepper

4 center-cut lamb
   loin chops (about
   4 ounces each),
   1 inch thick

2 cloves garlic, minced

**1.** Prepare grill for direct cooking or preheat broiler.

**2.** Combine oil, cumin, coriander, salt, cinnamon and red pepper in small bowl; mix well. Rub spice mixture over both sides of lamb chops. Sprinkle with garlic.

**3.** Grill lamb, covered, or broil 4 to 5 inches from heat about 5 minutes per side for medium or until desired doneness.

# GREEK LEG OF LAMB

Makes 6 to 8 servings

2½ to 3 pounds boneless leg of lamb

¼ cup Dijon mustard

2 tablespoons minced fresh rosemary leaves

2 teaspoons salt

2 teaspoons black pepper

4 cloves garlic, minced

¼ cup olive oil

**1.** Untie and unroll lamb to lie flat; trim fat.

**2.** Combine mustard, rosemary, salt, pepper and garlic in small bowl; whisk in oil until blended. Spread mixture evenly over lamb, coating both sides.

**3.** Place lamb in large resealable food storage bag. Seal bag; marinate in refrigerator at least 2 hours or overnight, turning several times.

**4.** Prepare grill for direct cooking. Grill lamb over medium-high heat 35 to 40 minutes or until desired doneness. Remove lamb to cutting board; tent with foil. Let stand 10 minutes before slicing. (Remove from grill at 140°F for medium. Temperature will rise 5°F while resting.)

# SPICY PORK AND VEGETABLE STEW

## Makes 6 servings

1 tablespoon olive oil

1½ pounds boneless pork loin, trimmed and cut into ½-inch pieces

2 red bell peppers, cut into ½-inch pieces

1 package (8 ounces) sliced mushrooms

1 cup chopped onion

1 medium butternut or acorn squash, peeled and cut into ½-inch pieces

1 can (about 14 ounces) diced tomatoes

1 can (about 14 ounces) chicken broth

1 teaspoon salt

½ teaspoon red pepper flakes

½ teaspoon dried thyme

½ teaspoon black pepper

Fresh oregano sprigs (optional)

**1.** Heat oil in large saucepan or Dutch oven over medium-high heat. Add pork in two batches; cook about 5 minutes or until browned, stirring occasionally.

**2.** Add bell peppers, mushrooms and onion to saucepan; cook and stir 5 minutes. Stir in squash, tomatoes, broth, salt, red pepper flakes, thyme and black pepper; bring to a boil over high heat. Reduce heat to low; cover and cook 1 hour or until pork is tender. Garnish with oregano.

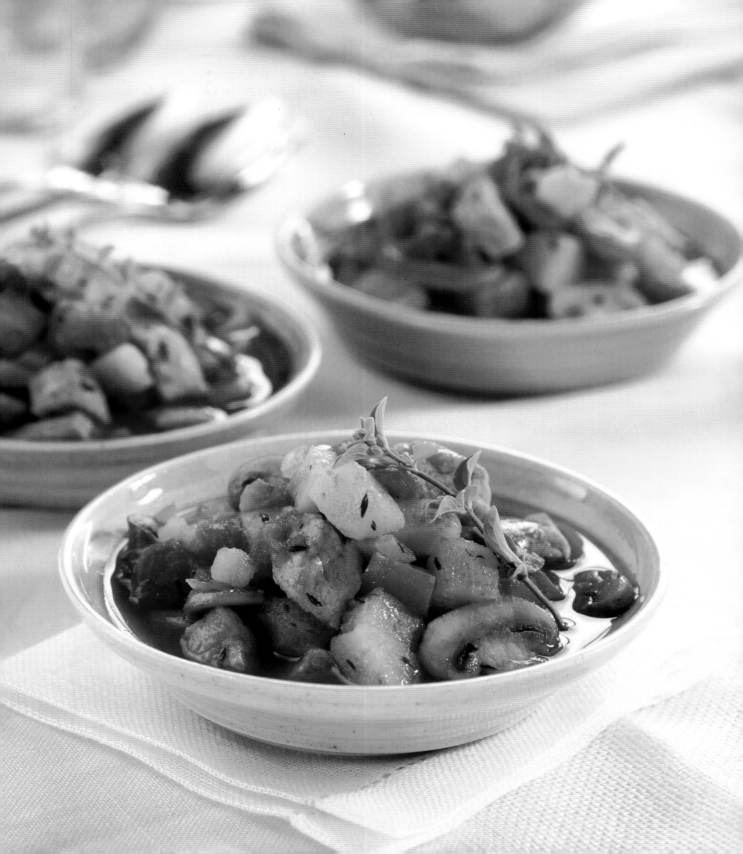

# PORK TENDERLOIN WITH AVOCADO-TOMATILLO SALSA

Makes 4 servings

1½ teaspoons chili powder

½ teaspoon ground cumin

½ teaspoon salt, divided

1 pound pork tenderloin

1 tablespoon olive oil

2 medium tomatillos, diced

½ ripe avocado, diced

2 tablespoons finely chopped red onion

1 to 2 tablespoons chopped fresh cilantro

1 tablespoon lime juice

1 jalapeño pepper,* seeded and finely chopped

1 clove garlic, minced

4 lime wedges (optional)

*Jalapeño peppers can sting and irritate the skin, so wear rubber gloves when handling peppers and do not touch your eyes.

**1.** Preheat oven to 425°F. Line baking sheet with foil.

**2.** Combine chili powder, cumin and ¼ teaspoon salt in small bowl; mix well. Sprinkle over all sides of pork, pressing to allow spices to adhere.

**3.** Heat oil in large nonstick skillet over medium-high heat. Add pork; cook 3 minutes or until browned. Turn and cook 2 to 3 minutes or until browned. Place on prepared baking sheet.

**4.** Roast 20 to 25 minutes or until pork is 145°F and barely pink in center. Remove pork to cutting board; tent with foil. Let stand 10 minutes before slicing.

**5.** Meanwhile, combine tomatillos, avocado, onion, cilantro, lime juice, jalapeño, garlic and remaining ¼ teaspoon salt; toss gently. Serve pork with salsa and lime wedges, if desired.

**TIP:** Choose firm tomatillos with dry husks that are not too ragged. Store in a paper bag in refrigerator for up to a month. Remove husks and wash tomatillos well before using.

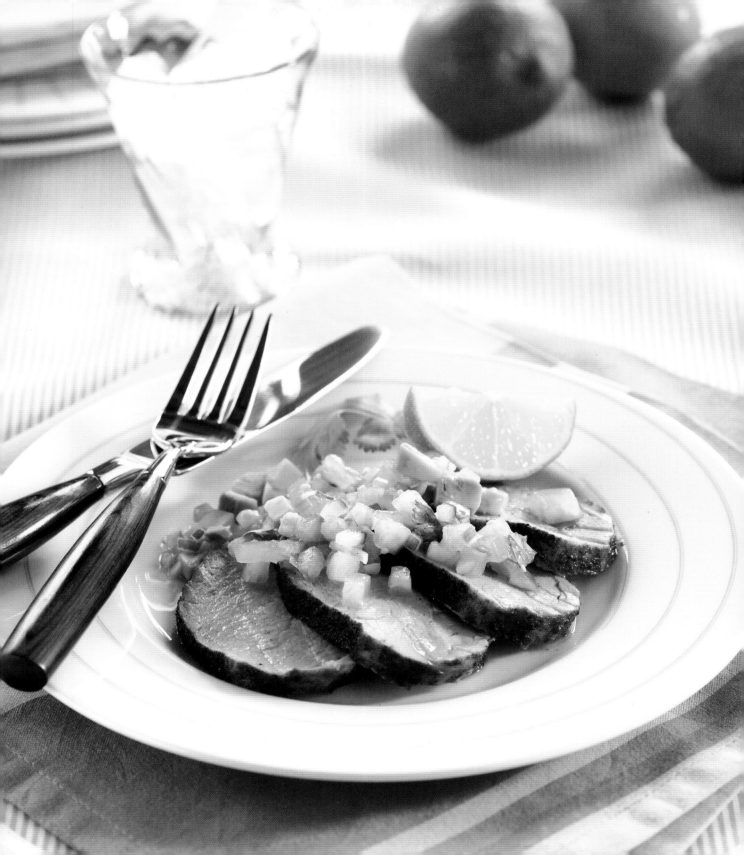

# SAUSAGE AND PEPPERS

Makes 4 servings

1 pound hot or mild Italian sausage links

2 tablespoons olive oil

3 medium onions, cut into ½-inch slices

2 red bell peppers, cut into ½-inch slices

2 green bell peppers, cut into ½-inch slices

1½ teaspoons coarse salt, divided

1 teaspoon dried oregano

**1.** Fill medium saucepan half full with water; bring to a boil over high heat. Add sausage; cook 5 minutes over medium heat. Drain and cut diagonally into 1-inch slices.

**2.** Heat oil in large cast iron skillet over medium-high heat. Add sausage; cook about 10 minutes or until browned, stirring occasionally. Remove sausage to plate; set aside.

**3.** Add onions, bell peppers, 1 teaspoon salt and oregano to skillet; cook over medium heat about 30 minutes or until vegetables are very soft and browned in spots, stirring occasionally.

**4.** Stir sausage and remaining ½ teaspoon salt into skillet; cook 3 minutes or until heated through.

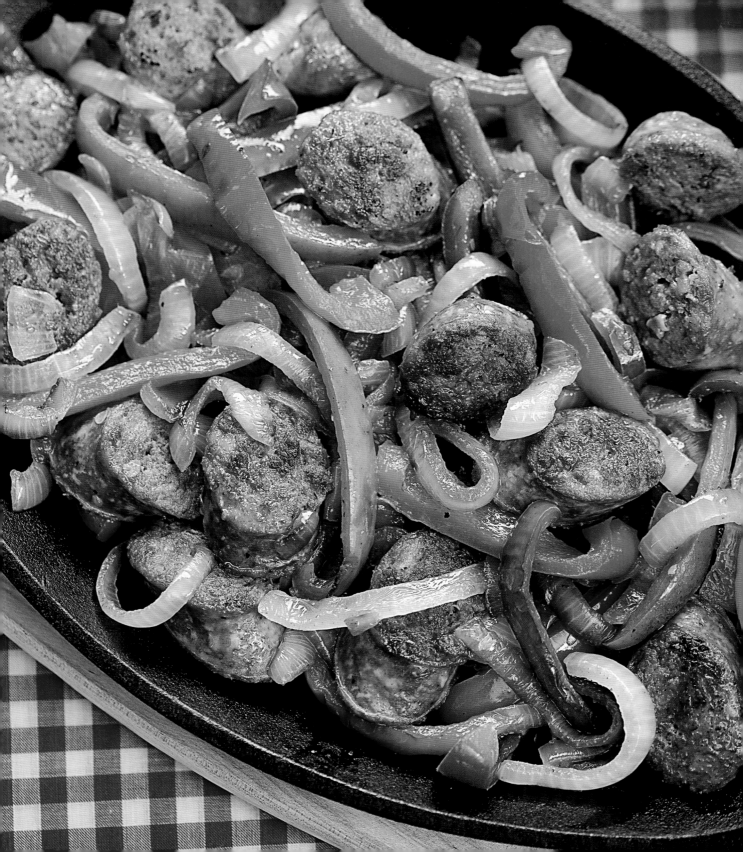

# PORK LOIN WITH CHILI-SPICE SAUCE

Makes 6 servings

1 cup chopped onion

¼ cup orange juice

2 cloves garlic

1 tablespoon cider vinegar

1½ teaspoons chili powder

1 teaspoon salt, divided

¼ teaspoon dried thyme

¼ teaspoon ground cumin

¼ teaspoon ground cinnamon

⅛ teaspoon ground allspice

⅛ teaspoon ground cloves

1 boneless pork loin roast (about 1½ pounds), trimmed

3 firm large bananas

2 limes

2 teaspoons coconut oil

1 ripe large papaya, peeled, seeded and cubed

1 green onion, minced

**1.** Preheat oven to 350°F. Combine onion, orange juice and garlic in food processor; process until finely chopped. Pour into medium saucepan; stir in vinegar, chili powder, ¾ teaspoon salt, thyme, cumin, cinnamon, allspice and cloves. Cook over medium-high heat about 5 minutes or until thickened, stirring occasionally.

**2.** Cut ¼-inch-deep lengthwise slits down top and bottom of pork at 1½-inch intervals. Spread about 1 tablespoon spice paste over bottom; place pork in shallow roasting pan. Spread remaining 2 tablespoons spice paste over sides and top of pork, working mixture into slits.

**3.** Cover pork and roast 45 minutes or until 140°F. Remove from oven; pour off and discard liquid. *Increase oven temperature to 450°F.* Roast, uncovered, 10 minutes or until pork is browned and internal temperature reaches 145°F. Remove pork to cutting board; tent with foil. Let stand 10 minutes before slicing.

**4.** Meanwhile, peel bananas; cut diagonally into ½-inch-thick slices. Place in 9-inch pie plate or cake pan. Squeeze juice from one lime over bananas; drizzle with oil and toss to coat. Cover and bake at 450°F 4 minutes or until hot. Stir in papaya, juice of remaining lime, remaining ¼ teaspoon salt and green onion. Serve with pork.

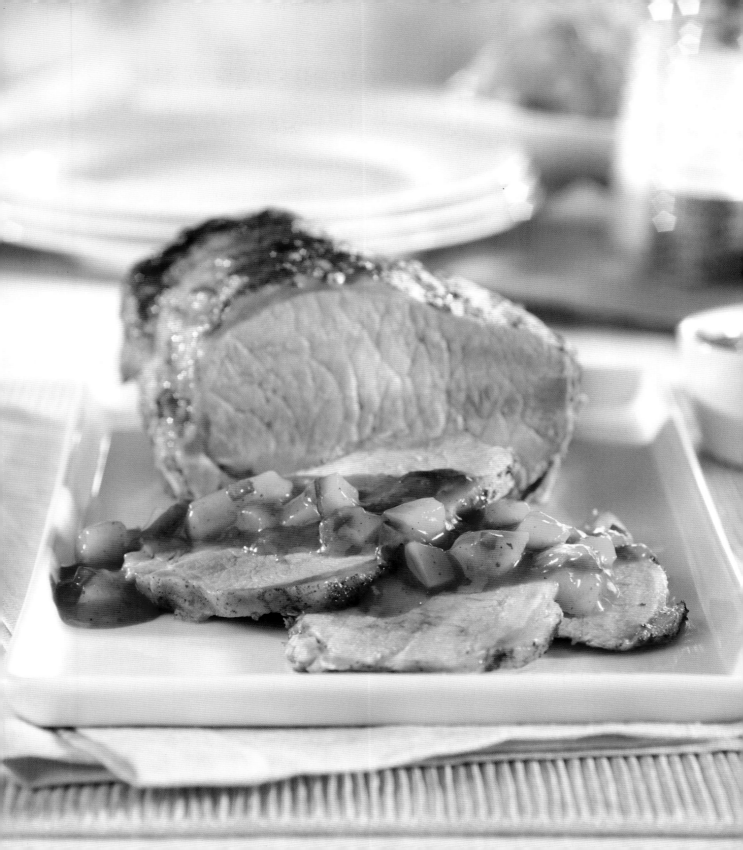

# ORANGE AND ROSEMARY BRAISED LAMB SHANKS

Makes 4 servings

## Dry Rub

1 teaspoon coarse salt

1 teaspoon dried oregano

1 teaspoon ground paprika

½ teaspoon black pepper

½ teaspoon ground cumin

⅛ teaspoon ground cloves

## Lamb

4 lamb shanks (about 1 pound each)

2 tablespoons olive oil

1 large leek, cut into ½-inch pieces

2 carrots, cut into 1-inch pieces

2 stalks celery, cut into 1-inch pieces

1 medium bulb fennel, cut into ¼-inch slices

½ cup dry red wine

4 cups chicken broth

1 orange, cut into ¼-inch slices

2 bay leaves

1 small bunch fresh thyme (about 6 sprigs)

1 sprig fresh rosemary

½ teaspoon salt

¼ teaspoon black pepper

**1.** Combine salt, oregano, paprika, pepper, cumin and cloves in small bowl; mix well. Rub over sides of lamb shanks. Cover and refrigerate at least 1 hour or overnight.

**2.** Preheat oven to 350°F. Heat oil in Dutch oven over medium-high heat. Add leek; cook and stir 3 minutes or until translucent. Add carrots, celery and fennel; cook and stir 5 minutes. Add wine; cook until reduced to about 1 tablespoon.

**3.** Arrange lamb on top of vegetables. Add broth, orange slices, bay leaves, thyme and rosemary. If broth does not cover lamb, add just enough water to cover. Bring to a boil; remove from heat.

**4.** Cover and bake 1½ to 2 hours or until lamb is very tender and meat begins to fall off the bone. Remove lamb and vegetables to platter; tent with foil. Discard herbs.

**5.** Skim fat from liquid in Dutch oven. Cook over medium heat 15 to 20 minutes or until liquid is reduced by half. Stir in salt and pepper. Serve sauce with lamb and vegetables.

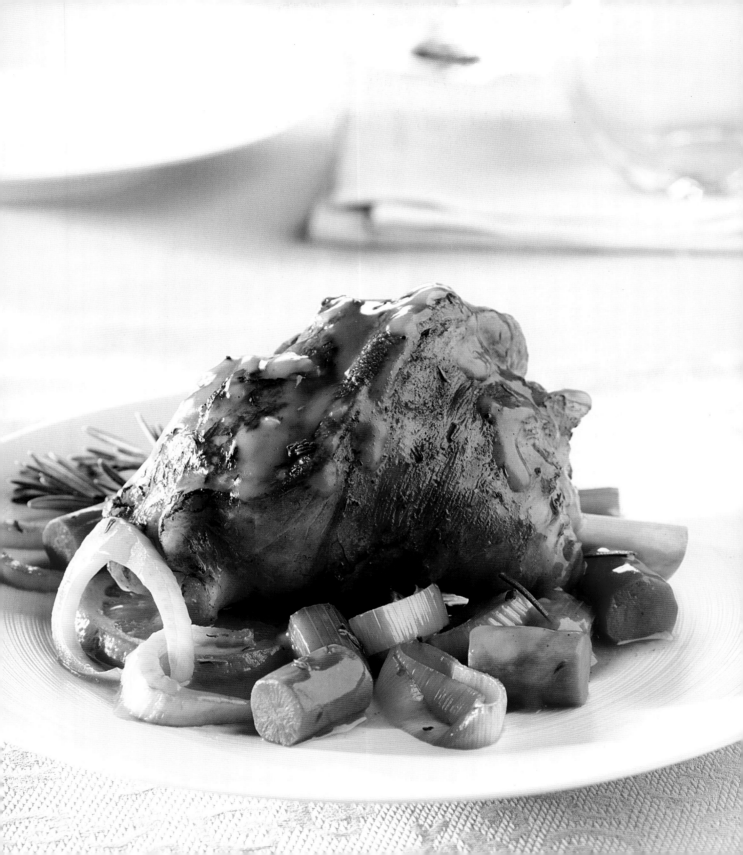

# CIDER PORK AND ONIONS
## Makes 8 servings

2 to 3 tablespoons olive oil

4 to 4½ pounds bone-in pork shoulder roast (pork butt)

4 to 5 medium onions, sliced (about 4 cups)

1 teaspoon salt, divided

4 cloves garlic, minced

3 sprigs fresh rosemary

½ teaspoon black pepper

2 to 3 cups apple cider

**1.** Preheat oven to 325°F. Heat 2 tablespoons oil in Dutch oven over medium-high heat. Add pork; cook until browned on all sides. Remove to large plate.

**2.** Add onions and ½ teaspoon salt to Dutch oven; cook and stir 10 minutes or until translucent, adding additional oil as needed to prevent burning. Add garlic; cook and stir 1 minute. Add pork and rosemary; sprinkle with remaining ½ teaspoon salt and pepper. Add cider to come about halfway up sides of pork.

**3.** Cover and bake 2 to 2½ hours or until very tender. (Meat should be almost falling off the bones.) Remove pork to platter; tent with foil.

**4.** Remove and discard rosemary sprigs. Boil liquid in Dutch oven over medium-high heat about 20 minutes or until reduced by half; skim fat. Season with additional salt and pepper, if desired. Cut pork; serve with sauce.

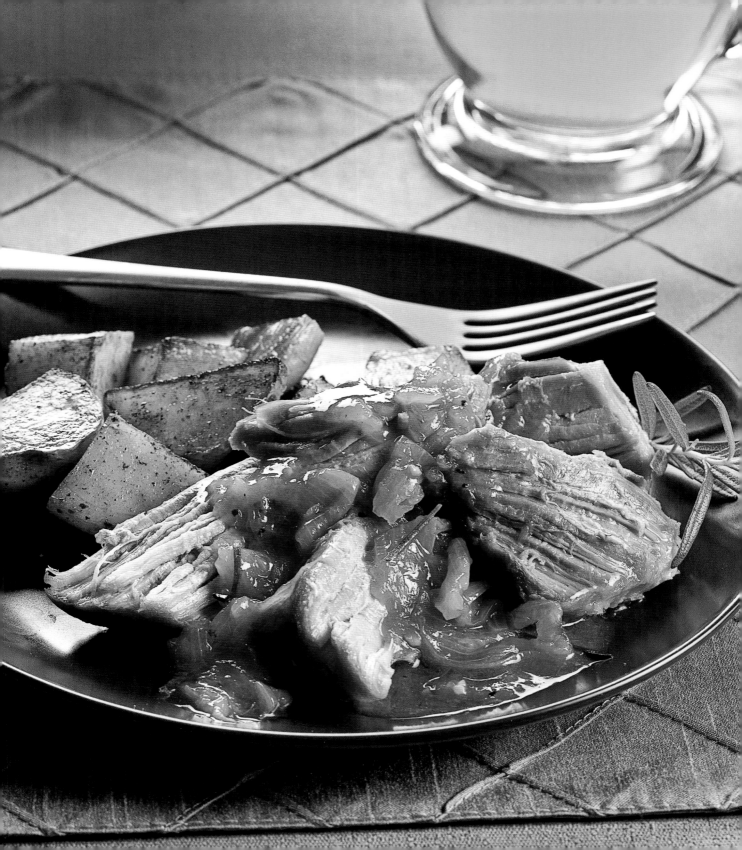

# PORK WITH APPLES, FENNEL AND CABBAGE

Makes 4 servings

1 cup apple cider, divided

2 tablespoons balsamic vinegar

½ teaspoon caraway seeds

½ teaspoon dried thyme

4 boneless pork chops (about 4 ounces each)

¼ teaspoon salt

¼ teaspoon black pepper

1 tablespoon olive oil

3 cups sliced green cabbage

1 medium bulb fennel, cut into ¼-inch slices

1 small onion, cut into ¼-inch slices

1 large apple, thinly sliced

2 teaspoons arrowroot or tapioca starch

**1.** Combine ⅔ cup cider, vinegar, caraway seeds and thyme in small bowl; mix well.

**2.** Sprinkle pork chops with salt and pepper. Heat oil in large nonstick skillet over medium-high heat. Add pork; cook 2 to 3 minutes per side or until lightly browned. Remove to plate.

**3.** Add cabbage, fennel, onion and apple cider mixture to skillet. Reduce heat to medium-low; cover and cook 15 minutes, stirring occasionally.

**4.** Return pork chops and any accumulated juices to skillet. Add apple; cover and cook 5 minutes or until pork chops are barely pink in center. Use slotted spoon to transfer pork, apple and vegetables to plate; tent with foil. Measure juices from skillet; add water to equal 1 cup. Return to skillet.

**5.** Stir remaining ⅓ cup apple cider into arrowroot in small bowl until smooth. Slowly add mixture to skillet; cook and stir over low heat just until sauce thickens. Serve over pork and vegetables.

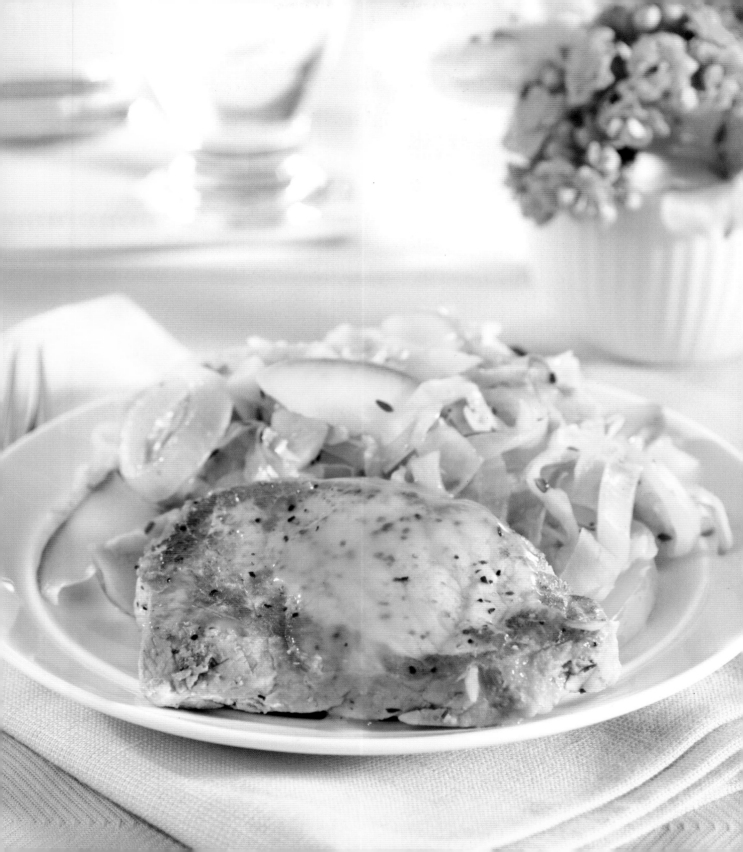

# HOMEMADE SAUSAGE PATTIES

Makes 16 sausage patties

1½ **pounds ground pork**

½ **pound ground turkey**

2 **teaspoons
ground sage**

1½ **teaspoons salt**

1 **to 1½ teaspoons
black pepper**

1 **teaspoon
dried thyme**

½ **teaspoon whole
fennel seeds,
crushed (optional)**

**1.** Combine pork, turkey, sage, salt, pepper, thyme and fennel seeds, if desired, in large bowl; mix well. Cover and refrigerate at least 1 hour or up to 24 hours.

**2.** For each sausage patty, shape ¼ cup pork mixture into ½-inch-thick patty about 2½ inches in diameter.

**3.** Heat large skillet over medium-high heat. Add as many sausage patties as will fit in single layer without crowding skillet. Cook sausage 2 minutes; turn and cook 2 minutes.

**4.** Reduce heat to medium-low; cook sausage 3 to 4 minutes per side or until no longer pink in center. Repeat with remaining sausage patties.

**NOTE:** Sausage patties can be wrapped tightly with plastic wrap and frozen up to 1 month.

# DELUXE MEDITERRANEAN LAMB BURGERS

Makes 4 servings

1½ pounds ground lamb

1 tablespoon minced garlic

2 teaspoons Greek seasoning

1 teaspoon paprika

½ teaspoon salt, divided

½ teaspoon black pepper

4 thin slices red onion, separated into rings

1 tablespoon olive oil

1 teaspoon chopped fresh mint or parsley

1 teaspoon red wine vinegar

Spinach leaves

4 to 8 slices tomatoes

**1.** Oil grid. Prepare grill for direct cooking.

**2.** Combine lamb, garlic, Greek seasoning, paprika, ¼ teaspoon salt and pepper in large bowl; mix gently. Shape into four patties about ¾ inch thick. Cover and refrigerate.

**3.** Combine onion, oil, mint, vinegar and remaining ¼ teaspoon salt in small bowl; mix well.

**4.** Grill patties, covered, over medium heat 8 to 10 minutes (or uncovered 13 to 15 minutes) until cooked through (160°F) or until desired doneness, turning occasionally.

**5.** Serve burgers over spinach; top with tomatoes and onion mixture.

# PORK TENDERLOIN WITH PLUM SALSA

Makes 4 servings

2 to 3 limes

Plum Salsa
(recipe follows)

1 pork tenderloin
(about 1 pound)

⅓ cup coconut aminos

1 tablespoon dark
sesame oil

2 cloves garlic, minced

2 tablespoons honey

Fresh cilantro sprigs
(optional)

**1.** Juice limes into measuring cup. Measure 2 tablespoons for marinade; set aside. Prepare Plum Salsa using remaining juice.

**2.** Place pork in large resealable food storage bag. Combine coconut aminos, 2 tablespoons lime juice, oil and garlic in small bowl; mix well. Pour over pork. Seal bag; turn to coat. Marinate in refrigerator overnight, turning occasionally.

**3.** Preheat oven to 375°F. Drain pork; reserve 2 tablespoons marinade. Combine reserved marinade and honey in small saucepan; bring to a boil over medium-high heat. Cook 1 minute, stirring once.

**4.** To ensure even cooking, tuck narrow end of tenderloin under roast, forming even thickness of meat. Secure with kitchen string. Place pork on rack in shallow roasting pan. Brush with some of honey mixture.

**5.** Roast 15 minutes; brush with remaining honey mixture. Roast 10 minutes or until 145°F. Remove pork to cutting board; tent with foil. Let stand 10 minutes before slicing.

**6.** Remove string from pork. Slice pork; serve with salsa. Garnish with cilantro sprigs.

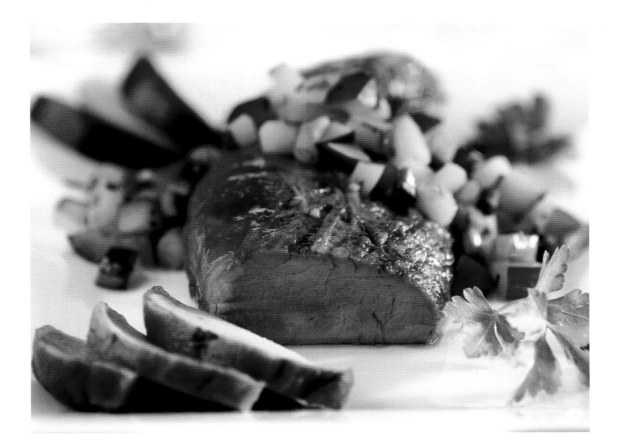

## PLUM SALSA

Makes 1 cup

2 cups coarsely
  chopped red plums
  (about 3)

2 tablespoons chopped
  green onion

2 tablespoons honey

1 tablespoon chopped
  fresh cilantro

2 teaspoons lime juice

Dash ground
  red pepper

Combine all ingredients in small bowl; mix well.
Cover and refrigerate at least 2 hours.

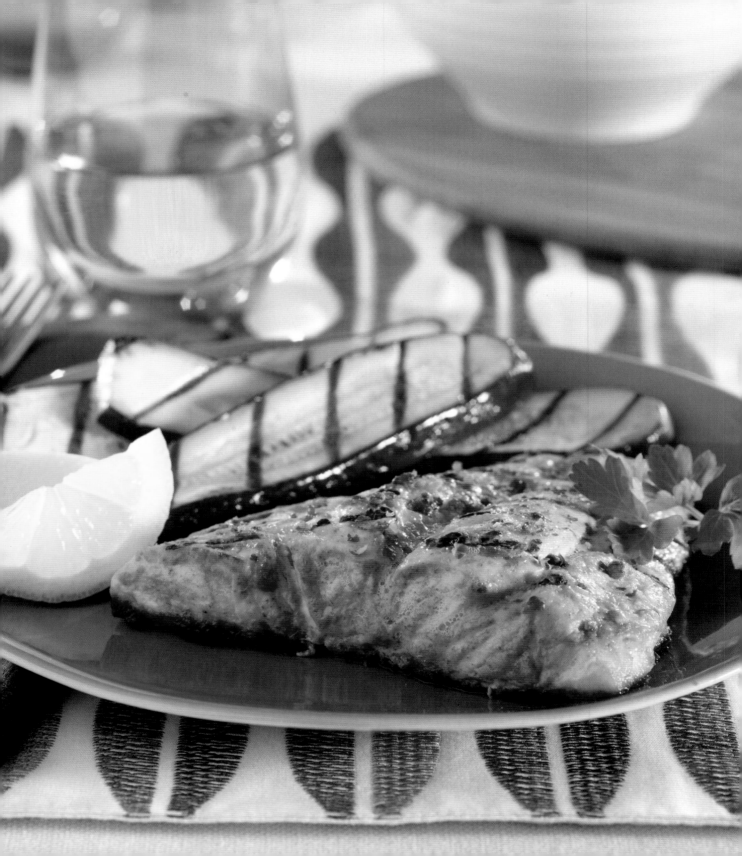

# FISH

## MUSTARD-GRILLED RED SNAPPER

### Makes 4 servings

½ cup Dijon mustard

1 tablespoon red wine vinegar

1 teaspoon ground red pepper

¼ teaspoon salt

4 red snapper fillets (about 6 ounces each)

**1.** Oil grid. Prepare grill for direct cooking.

**2.** Combine mustard, vinegar, red pepper and salt in small bowl; mix well. Coat snapper thoroughly with mustard mixture.

**3.** Grill fish, covered, over medium-high heat 4 minutes per side or until fish begins to flake when tested with fork.

# TERIYAKI SALMON

Makes 4 servings

⅓ cup coconut aminos

¼ cup honey

1 tablespoon white wine vinegar or balsamic vinegar

1 tablespoon grated fresh ginger

3 cloves garlic, minced

½ teaspoon dark sesame oil

Pinch red pepper flakes

4 salmon fillets (7 to 8 ounces each)

2 tablespoons minced green onion

Lime slices (optional)

**1.** Combine coconut aminos, honey, vinegar, ginger, garlic, sesame oil and red pepper flakes in medium bowl; mix well. Reserve ¼ cup marinade; set aside.

**2.** Place salmon in large resealable food storage bag; pour remaining marinade over fish. Seal bag; turn to coat. Marinate in refrigerator 1 to 2 hours, turning occasionally.

**3.** Oil grid. Prepare grill for direct cooking or preheat broiler. Remove fish from marinade; discard marinade.

**4.** Grill or broil 8 to 10 minutes or until fish begins to flake when tested with fork. (To broil, place fish on oiled foil-lined baking sheet.) Brush with reserved marinade; sprinkle with green onion. Garnish with lime slices.

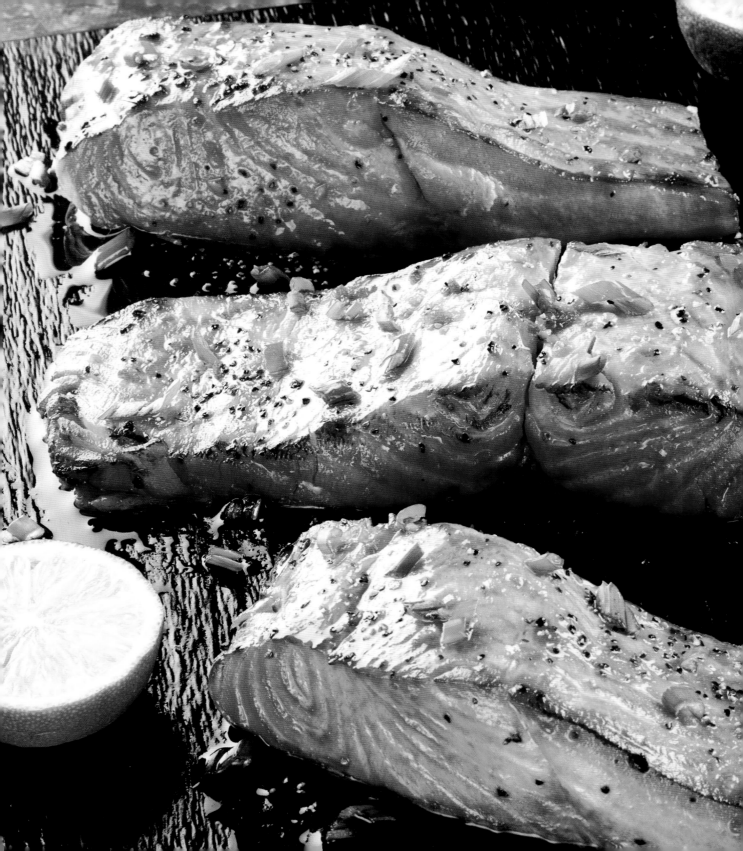

# HALIBUT WITH TOMATO AND BROCCOLI SAUCE

Makes 4 servings

2 tablespoons olive oil

2 cups chopped
   fresh broccoli

2½ cups diced fresh
   tomatoes

2 tablespoons
   lemon juice

1 tablespoon
   chopped garlic

1 tablespoon chopped
   fresh tarragon *or*
   1 teaspoon dried
   tarragon

½ teaspoon salt

½ teaspoon black
   pepper

4 halibut steaks
   (4 ounces each)

   Lemon wedges
   (optional)

**1.** Heat oil in large skillet over medium heat. Add broccoli; cook and stir 5 minutes. Add tomatoes, lemon juice, garlic, tarragon, salt and pepper; cook and stir 5 minutes.

**2.** Add halibut to skillet; cover and cook 10 minutes or until fish begins to flake when tested with fork.

**3.** Divide vegetables evenly among four plates; top with fish. Serve with lemon wedges, if desired.

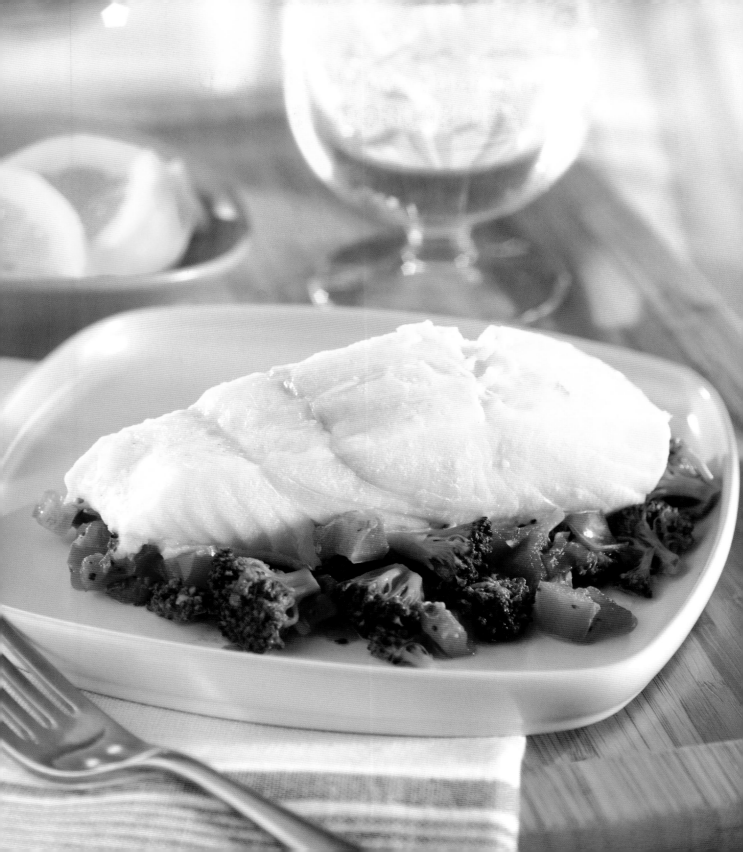

# CAJUN BLACKENED TUNA

Makes 4 servings

1½ teaspoons garlic salt

1 teaspoon paprika

1 teaspoon dried thyme or oregano

½ teaspoon ground cumin

¼ teaspoon ground red pepper

⅛ teaspoon white pepper

⅛ teaspoon black pepper

2 tablespoons butter, melted

4 tuna steaks (6 ounces each), 1 inch thick

Lemon wedges

**1.** Prepare grill for direct cooking or heat grill pan or skillet over medium-high heat.

**2.** Combine garlic salt, paprika, thyme, cumin, red pepper, white pepper and black pepper in small bowl; mix well. Brush butter over both sides of tuna; sprinkle with spice mixture.

**3.** Grill fish over medium-high heat 2 to 3 minutes per side for medium rare. Serve with lemon wedges.

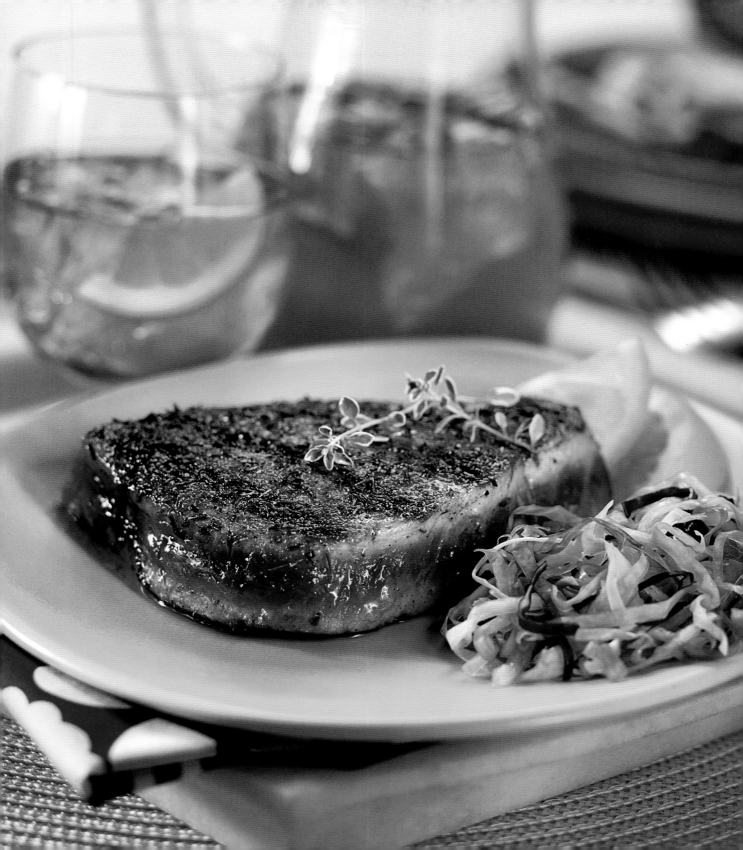

# DILLED SALMON IN PARCHMENT

## Makes 2 servings

2 skinless salmon fillets (4 to 6 ounces each)

2 tablespoons butter, melted

1 tablespoon lemon juice

1 tablespoon chopped fresh dill

1 tablespoon chopped shallots

Salt and black pepper

**1.** Preheat oven to 400°F. Cut two pieces of parchment paper into 12-inch squares; fold squares in half diagonally and cut into half heart shapes. Open parchment; place salmon on one side of each heart.

**2.** Combine butter and lemon juice in small bowl; drizzle over fish. Sprinkle with dill, shallots and salt and pepper to taste.

**3.** Fold parchment hearts in half. Beginning at top of heart, fold edges together, 2 inches at a time. At tip of heart, fold parchment over to seal. Place parchment packets on baking sheet.

**4.** Bake about 10 minutes or until parchment packet puffs up. To serve, cut an "X" through top layer of parchment and fold back points to display contents.

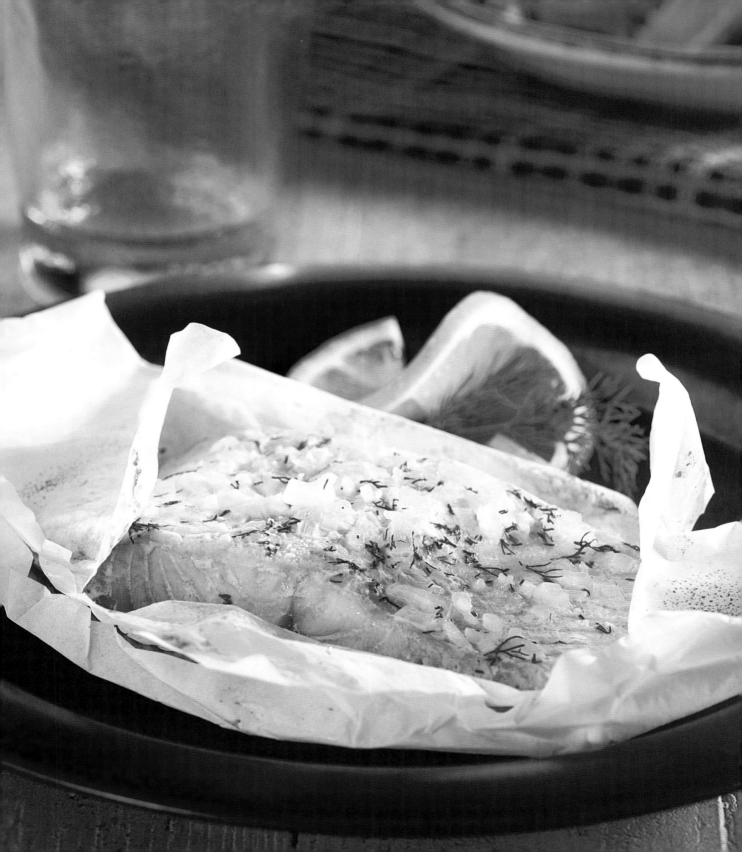

# GROUPER SCAMPI

Makes 4 servings

3 tablespoons butter, softened

1 tablespoon dry white wine

1½ teaspoons minced garlic

½ teaspoon grated lemon peel

⅛ teaspoon black pepper

1½ pounds grouper, red snapper or orange roughy fillets (4 to 5 ounces each)

**1.** Preheat oven to 450°F. Line shallow baking pan with foil.

**2.** Combine butter, wine, garlic, lemon peel and pepper in small bowl; mix well. Place fish in prepared pan; top with seasoned butter.

**3.** Bake 10 to 12 minutes or until fish begins to flake when tested with fork.

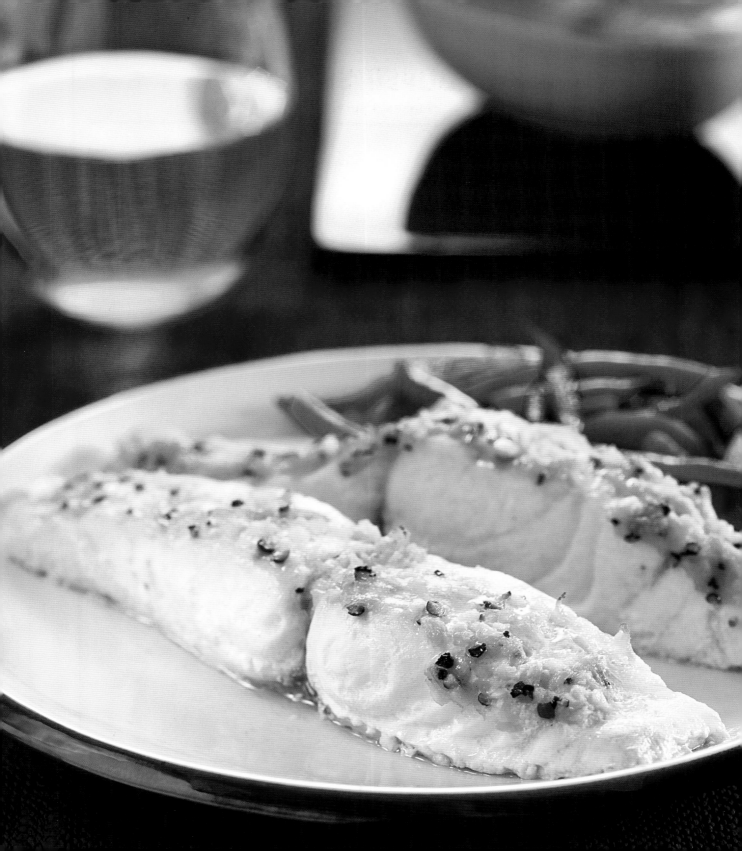

# SZECHUAN TUNA STEAKS

Makes 4 servings

4 tuna steaks
  (6 ounces each),
  1 inch thick

¼ cup dry sherry

¼ cup coconut aminos

1 tablespoon dark
  sesame oil

1 clove garlic, minced

¼ teaspoon red
  pepper flakes

3 tablespoons
  chopped fresh
  cilantro (optional)

**1.** Place tuna in large shallow glass dish. Combine sherry, coconut aminos, sesame oil, garlic and red pepper flakes in small bowl; mix well. Reserve ¼ cup sherry mixture for serving; set aside.

**2.** Pour remaining sherry mixture over fish; cover and marinate in refrigerator 40 minutes, turning once.

**3.** Oil grid. Prepare grill for direct cooking. Drain fish; discard marinade.

**4.** Grill over medium-high heat 3 minutes per side or until seared. (Fish should feel somewhat soft in center.*) Remove fish to cutting board; cut each steak into thin slices. Drizzle with reserved sherry mixture; garnish with cilantro.

*Tuna becomes dry and tough if overcooked. Cook to medium doneness for best results.*

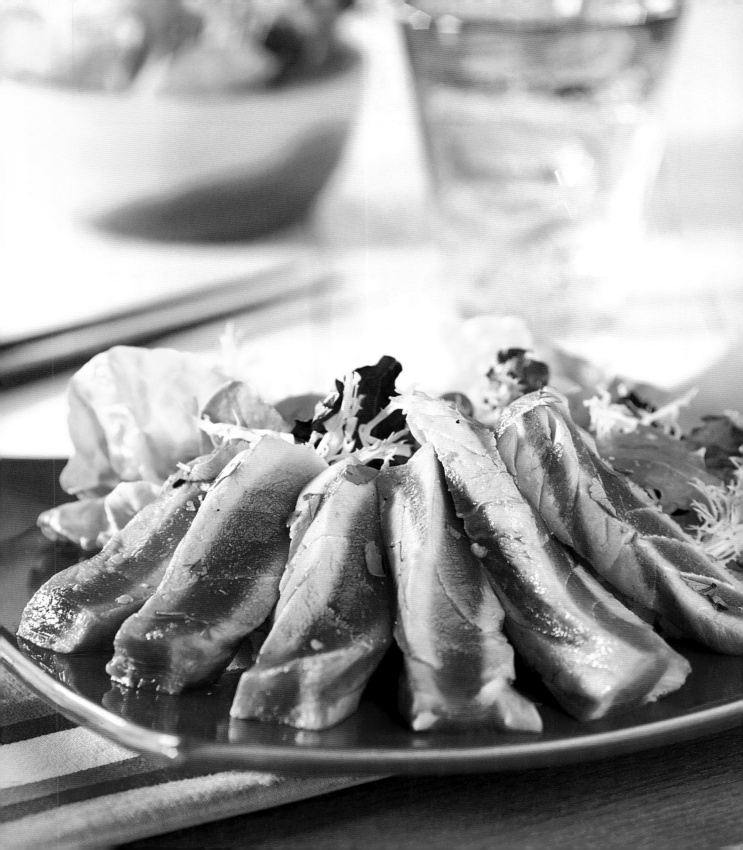

# GREEK-STYLE SALMON

Makes 4 servings

1½ tablespoons olive oil

1¾ cups diced tomatoes, drained

¼ cup pitted black olives, coarsely chopped

¼ cup pitted green olives, coarsely chopped

3 tablespoons lemon juice

2 tablespoons chopped fresh Italian parsley

1 tablespoon capers, rinsed and drained

2 medium cloves garlic, thinly sliced

¼ teaspoon black pepper

4 salmon fillets (4 to 6 ounces each)

**1.** Heat oil in large skillet over medium heat. Add tomatoes, olives, lemon juice, parsley, capers, garlic and pepper; bring to a simmer, stirring frequently. Cook 5 minutes or until reduced by about one third, stirring occasionally.

**2.** Rinse salmon and pat dry with paper towels. Push sauce to one side of skillet. Add fish to skillet; spoon sauce over fish.

**3.** Cover and cook 10 to 15 minutes or until fish begins to flake when tested with fork.

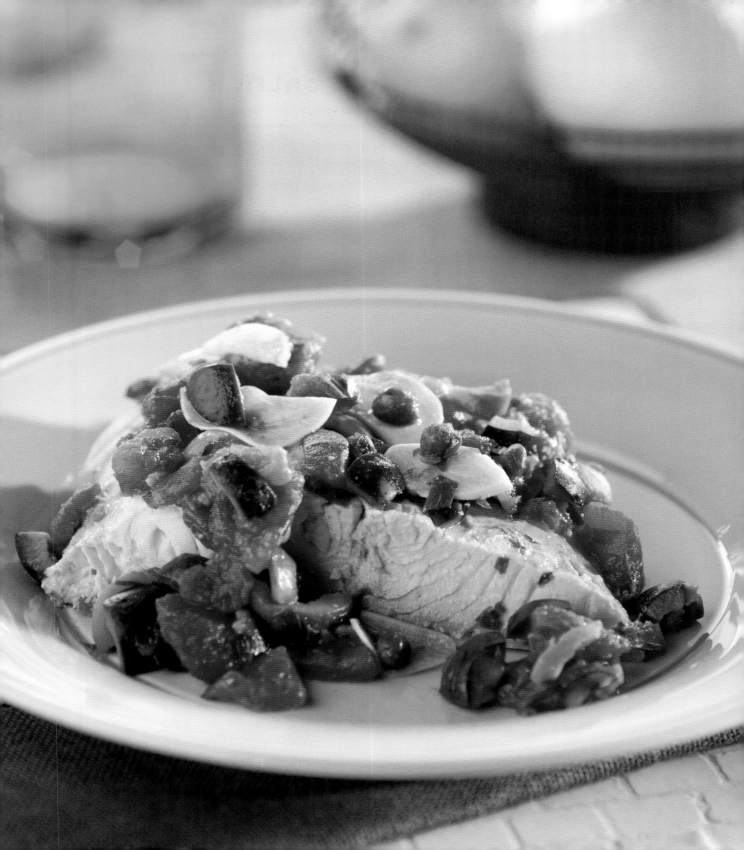

# BROILED TROUT WITH PINE NUT BUTTER

Makes 4 servings

¼ cup olive oil

¼ cup dry white wine

2 tablespoons minced fresh chives

2 tablespoons chopped fresh parsley

½ teaspoon salt

⅛ teaspoon black pepper

4 whole trout (about 8 ounces each), cleaned

¼ cup (½ stick) butter, softened

¼ cup pine nuts, finely chopped

Lemon wedges (optional)

**1.** Combine oil, wine, chives, parsley, salt and pepper in small bowl; mix well. Place trout in large resealable food storage bag. Pour marinade over fish. Seal bag; turn to coat. Marinate in refrigerator 30 minutes or up to 2 hours, turning occasionally.

**2.** Combine butter and pine nuts in small bowl; mix well. Cover and let stand at room temperature until ready to use.

**3.** Preheat broiler. Line baking sheet or broiler pan with foil. Remove fish from marinade; reserve marinade. Place fish on prepared baking sheet.

**4.** Broil 4 to 6 inches from heat 4 minutes. Turn fish; brush with reserved marinade. Broil 4 to 6 minutes or until fish begins to flake when tested with fork. Discard remaining marinade.

**5.** Top each fish with dollop of butter mixture. Serve with lemon wedges, if desired.

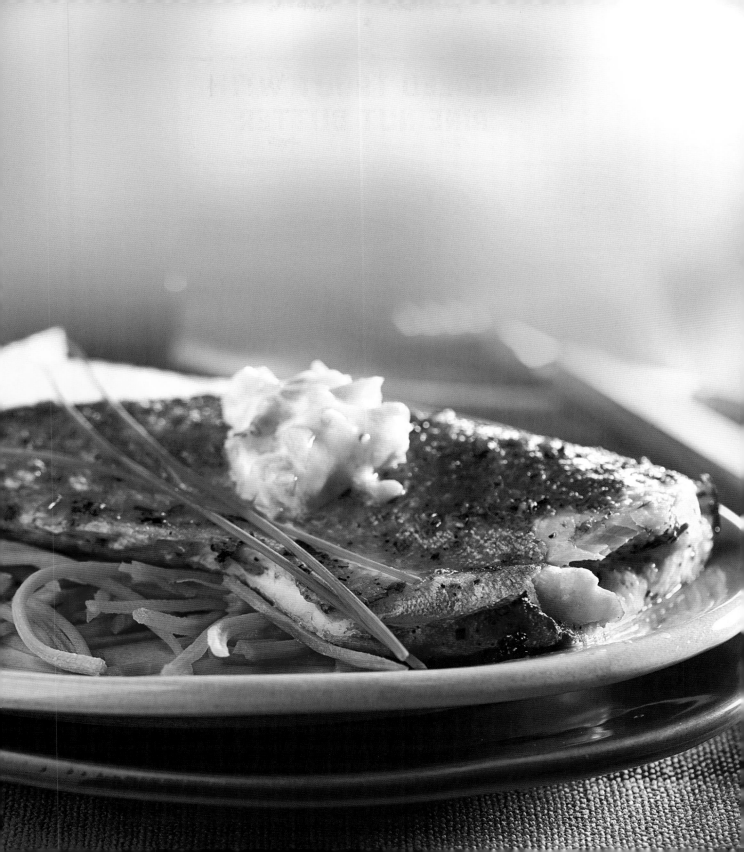

# BAKED ORANGE ROUGHY
# WITH VEGETABLES

Makes 2 servings

2 orange roughy fillets (4 to 6 ounces each)

1 tablespoon olive oil

1 medium carrot, cut into matchstick-size pieces

4 medium mushrooms, sliced

⅓ cup chopped onion

¼ cup chopped green or yellow bell pepper

1 clove garlic, minced

¼ teaspoon salt

Black pepper

Lemon wedges

**1.** Preheat oven to 350°F. Place orange roughy in shallow baking dish.

**2.** Bake 15 minutes or until fish begins to flake when tested with fork.

**3.** Meanwhile, heat oil in medium skillet over medium-high heat. Add carrot; cook 3 minutes, stirring occasionally. Add mushrooms, onion, bell pepper, garlic and salt; cook and stir 4 minutes or until vegetables are crisp-tender.

**4.** Serve vegetables over fish; sprinkle with black pepper. Serve with lemon wedges.

**NOTE:** To broil fish, place on rack of broiler pan. Broil 4 to 6 inches from heat 4 minutes per side or just until fish begins to flake when tested with fork.

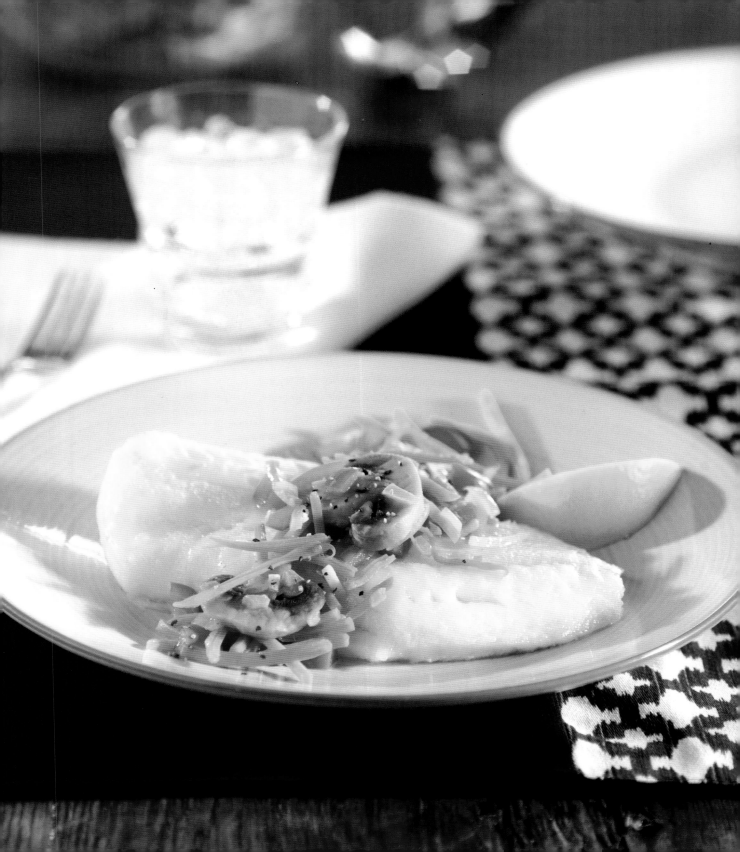

# ROASTED DILL SCROD WITH ASPARAGUS

Makes 4 servings

12 ounces asparagus spears, trimmed

1 tablespoon olive oil

4 scrod or cod fillets (about 5 ounces each)

1 tablespoon lemon juice

1 teaspoon dried dill weed

½ teaspoon salt

¼ teaspoon black pepper

Paprika (optional)

**1.** Preheat oven to 425°F.

**2.** Place asparagus in 13×9-inch baking dish; drizzle with oil. Roll asparagus to coat lightly with oil; push to edges of dish, stacking asparagus into two layers.

**3.** Arrange scrod in center of dish; drizzle with lemon juice. Combine dill weed, salt and pepper in small bowl; sprinkle over fish and asparagus. Sprinkle with paprika, if desired.

**4.** Roast 15 to 17 minutes or until asparagus is crisp-tender and fish begins to flake when tested with fork.

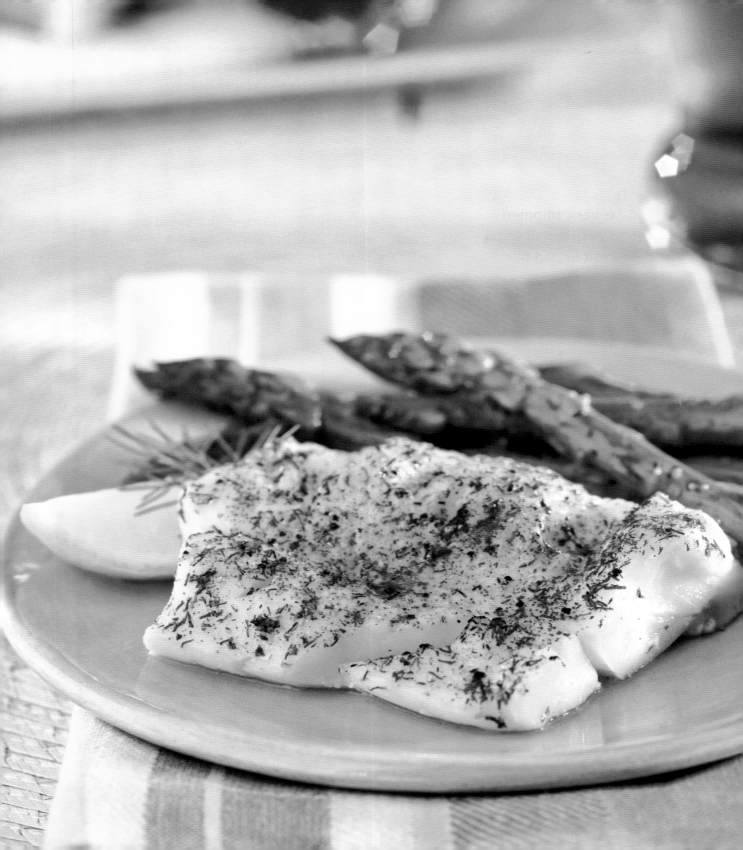

# GRILLED RED SNAPPER WITH AVOCADO-PAPAYA SALSA

Makes 4 servings

1 teaspoon ground coriander

1 teaspoon paprika

¾ teaspoon salt

⅛ to ¼ teaspoon ground red pepper

½ cup diced ripe avocado

½ cup diced ripe papaya

2 tablespoons chopped fresh cilantro

1 tablespoon lime juice

1 tablespoon olive oil

4 skinless red snapper or halibut fillets (5 to 7 ounces each)

Lime wedges

**1.** Oil grid. Prepare grill for direct cooking. Combine coriander, paprika, salt and red pepper in small bowl; mix well.

**2.** Combine avocado, papaya, cilantro, lime juice and ¼ teaspoon spice mixture in medium bowl; mix well.

**3.** Brush oil over snapper; sprinkle with remaining spice mixture.

**4.** Grill fish, covered, over medium-high heat about 5 minutes per side or until fish begins to flake when tested with fork. Serve with salsa and lime wedges.

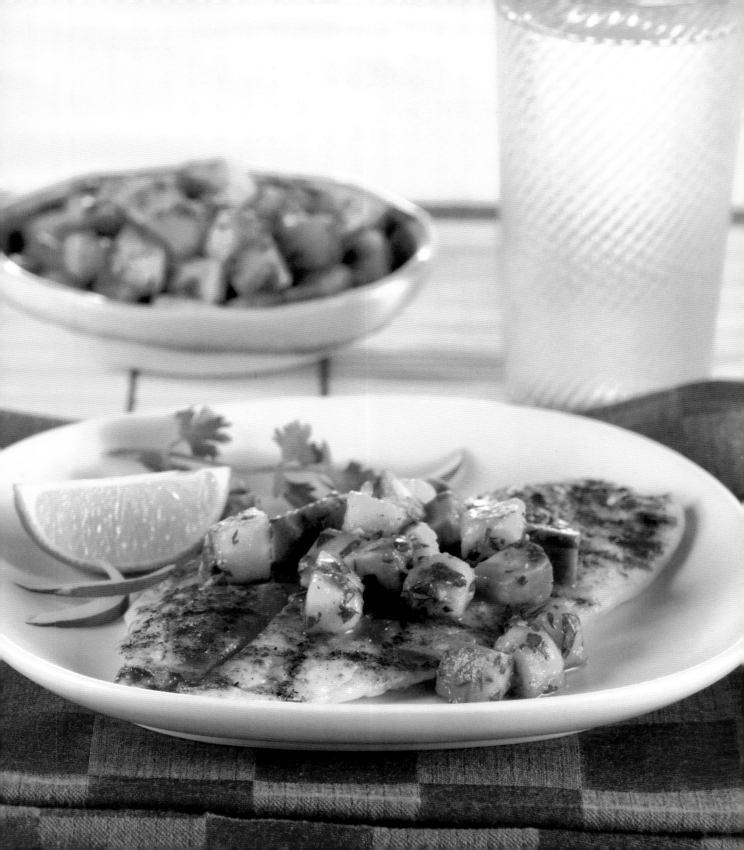

# SOUTHWESTERN TUNA SALAD

## Makes 4 servings

4 tuna steaks (about 4 ounces each)

Juice of 2 limes, divided

1½ tablespoons olive oil, divided

1 pint cherry or grape tomatoes, halved

¼ cup diced ripe avocado

1 jalapeño pepper,* seeded and minced

1 green onion, chopped

1 tablespoon chopped fresh cilantro

½ teaspoon salt

¼ teaspoon ground cumin

⅛ teaspoon black pepper

Lime wedges (optional)

*Jalapeño peppers can sting and irritate the skin, so wear rubber gloves when handling peppers and do not touch your eyes.

**1.** Place tuna in glass baking dish or shallow bowl; pour juice of one lime over fish. Marinate at room temperature 30 minutes, turning once.

**2.** Brush stovetop grill pan with ½ tablespoon oil; heat over medium heat. Add fish; cook 5 to 6 minutes per side. Remove to plate; cool to room temperature. Cut into bite-size pieces.

**3.** Combine tomatoes, avocado, jalapeño, green onion and cilantro in large bowl; mix well. Add fish.

**4.** Whisk remaining 1 tablespoon oil, lime juice, salt, cumin and black pepper in small bowl until well blended. Pour dressing over salad; toss gently to coat. Serve with lime wedges, if desired.

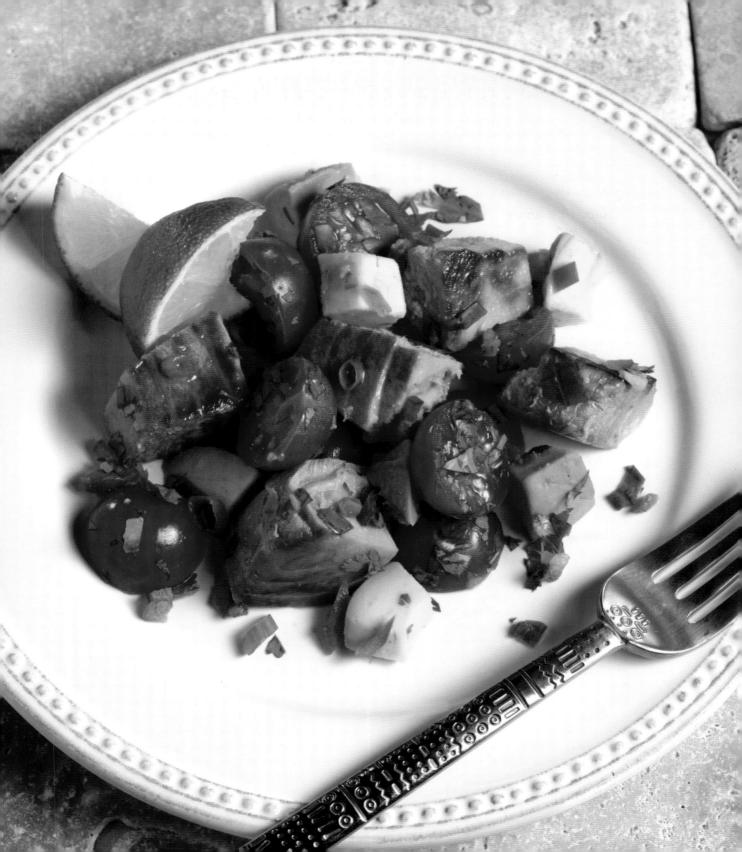

# GRILLED SWORDFISH SICILIAN STYLE

### Makes 4 to 6 servings

3 tablespoons extra virgin olive oil

1 clove garlic, minced

2 tablespoons lemon juice

¾ teaspoon salt

⅛ teaspoon black pepper

3 tablespoons capers, drained

1 tablespoon chopped fresh oregano or basil

4 swordfish steaks (about 6 ounces each), ¾ inch thick

**1.** Oil grid. Prepare grill for direct cooking.

**2.** Heat oil in small saucepan over low heat. Add garlic; cook 1 minute. Remove from heat; cool slightly. Whisk in lemon juice, salt and pepper until salt is dissolved. Stir in capers and oregano.

**3.** Grill fish over medium heat 3 to 4 minutes per side or until center is opaque. Serve with sauce.

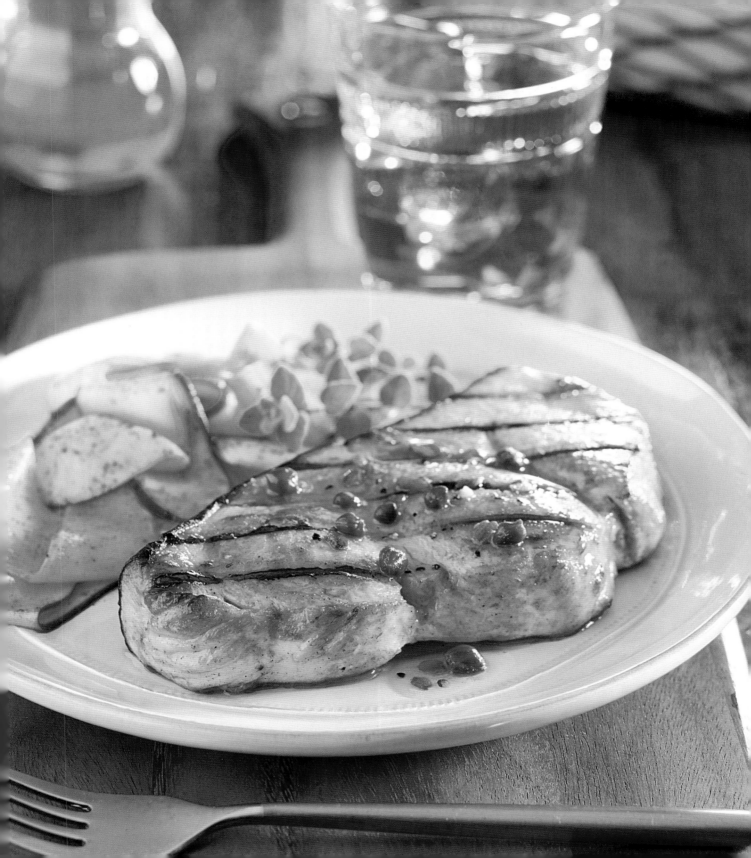

# BROILED COD WITH SALSA SALAD

Makes 4 servings

2 tablespoons olive oil, divided, plus additional for pan

2 medium tomatoes, chopped

1 green bell pepper, diced

1 serrano pepper,* minced

½ cup chopped red onion

1 tablespoon chopped fresh cilantro

1 teaspoon white wine vinegar

½ teaspoon salt, divided

½ teaspoon black pepper, divided

⅛ teaspoon dried oregano

4 cod fillets (3 to 4 ounces each), about ¾ inch thick

Lemon wedges

*Serrano peppers can sting and irritate the skin, so wear rubber gloves when handling peppers and do not touch your eyes.

**1.** Preheat broiler. Brush baking sheet with oil.

**2.** Combine tomatoes, bell pepper, serrano pepper, onion, cilantro, 1 tablespoon oil, vinegar, ¼ teaspoon salt and ¼ teaspoon black pepper in large bowl; mix well.

**3.** Combine remaining 1 tablespoon oil, ¼ teaspoon salt, ¼ teaspoon black pepper and oregano in small bowl; mix well. Place cod on prepared baking sheet; brush with oil mixture.

**4.** Broil 4 inches from heat source 6 to 8 minutes or until fish begins to flake when tested with fork. Serve with salad and lemon wedges.

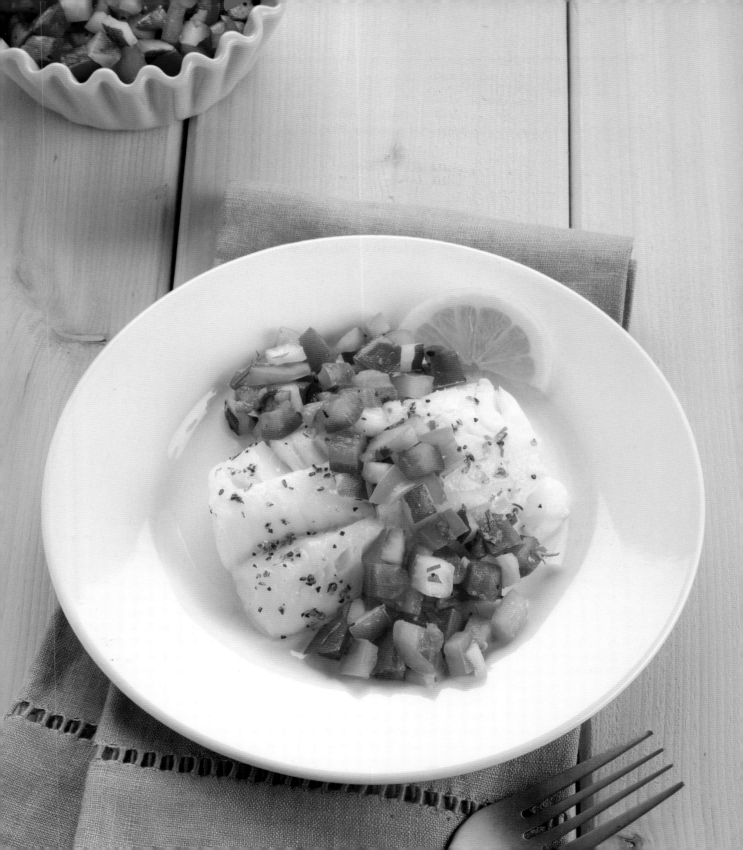

# MAPLE SALMON AND SWEETS

Makes 4 servings

½ cup maple syrup

2 tablespoons butter, melted

4 skin-on salmon fillets (4 to 6 ounces each)

2 medium sweet potatoes, peeled and cut into ¼-inch slices

1 teaspoon salt

¼ teaspoon black pepper

**1.** Combine maple syrup and butter in small bowl; mix well. Place salmon in large resealable food storage bag. Place sweet potatoes in another large resealable food storage bag. Pour half of syrup mixture into each bag. Seal bags; turn to coat. Marinate in refrigerator at least 2 hours or overnight, turning occasionally.

**2.** Oil grid. Prepare grill for direct cooking. Drain fish and sweet potatoes; discard marinade. Season with salt and pepper.

**3.** Grill salmon, skin side down, covered over medium heat 15 to 20 minutes or until fish begins to flake when tested with fork. (Do not turn.) Grill potatoes, covered, in single layer on grill topper 15 minutes or until tender and slightly browned, turning once or twice.

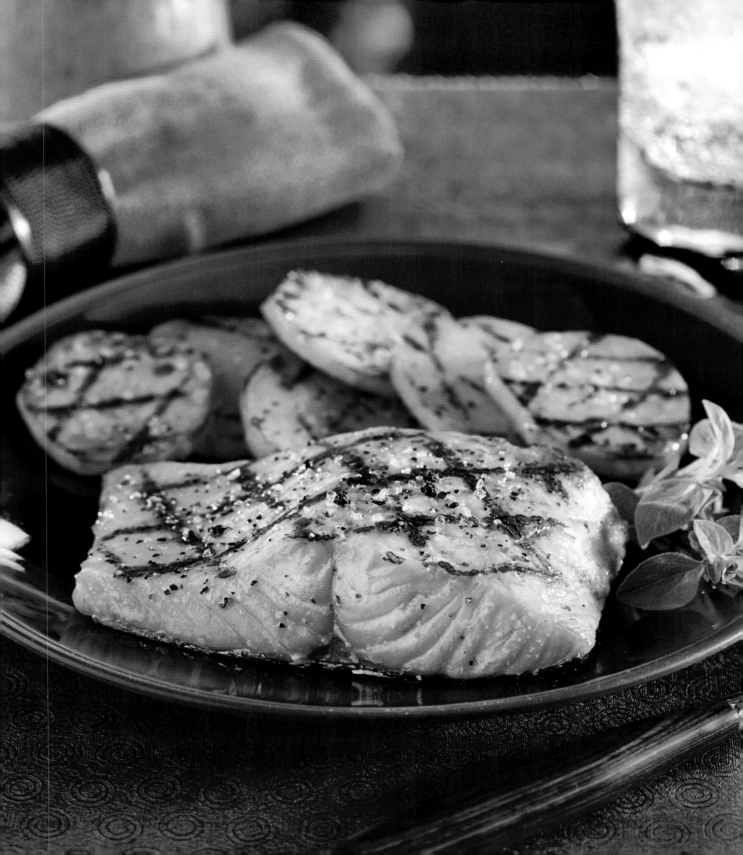

# PROSCIUTTO-WRAPPED SNAPPER

Makes 4 servings

2 tablespoons olive oil, divided

2 cloves garlic, minced

4 skinless red snapper or halibut fillets (6 to 7 ounces each)

½ teaspoon salt

½ teaspoon black pepper

8 large fresh sage leaves

8 thin slices prosciutto (4 ounces)

¼ cup dry marsala wine

**1.** Preheat oven to 400°F.

**2.** Combine 1 tablespoon oil and garlic in small bowl; brush over snapper. Sprinkle with salt and pepper. Place 2 sage leaves on each fillet. Wrap 2 slices prosciutto around fish to enclose sage leaves; tuck in ends of prosciutto.

**3.** Heat remaining 1 tablespoon oil in large ovenproof skillet over medium-high heat. Add fish, sage side down; cook 3 to 4 minutes or until prosciutto is crisp. Carefully turn fish.

**4.** Transfer skillet to oven; bake 8 to 10 minutes or until center is opaque. Remove fish to plate; tent with foil.

**5.** Add wine to skillet; cook over medium-high heat, scraping up browned bits from bottom of skillet. Cook 2 to 3 minutes or until liquid is reduced by half, stirring constantly. Drizzle over fish.

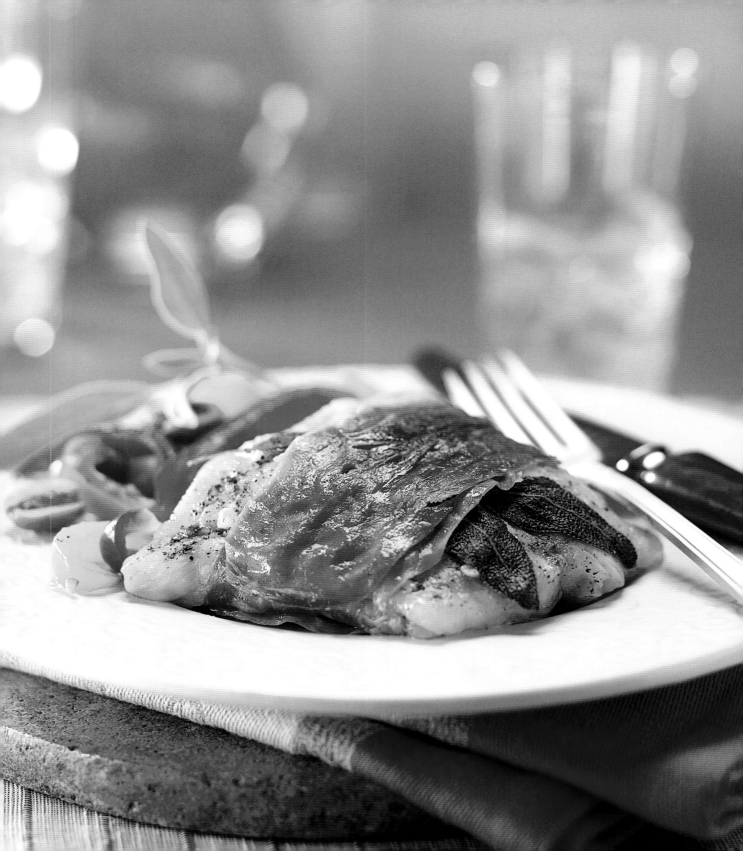

# TUNA STEAKS WITH PINEAPPLE AND TOMATO SALSA

Makes 4 servings

1 medium tomato, chopped

1 cup chopped fresh pineapple

2 tablespoons chopped fresh cilantro

1 jalapeño pepper,* seeded and minced

1 tablespoon minced red onion

2 teaspoons lime juice

½ teaspoon grated lime peel

4 tuna steaks (about 4 ounces each)

½ teaspoon salt

⅛ teaspoon black pepper

1 tablespoon olive oil

*Jalapeño peppers can sting and irritate the skin, so wear rubber gloves when handling peppers and do not touch your eyes.*

**1.** Combine tomato, pineapple, cilantro, jalapeño, onion, lime juice and lime peel in medium bowl; mix well.

**2.** Sprinkle tuna with salt and pepper. Heat oil in large nonstick skillet over medium-high heat. Add fish; cook 2 to 3 minutes per side for medium rare or until desired doneness. Serve with salsa.

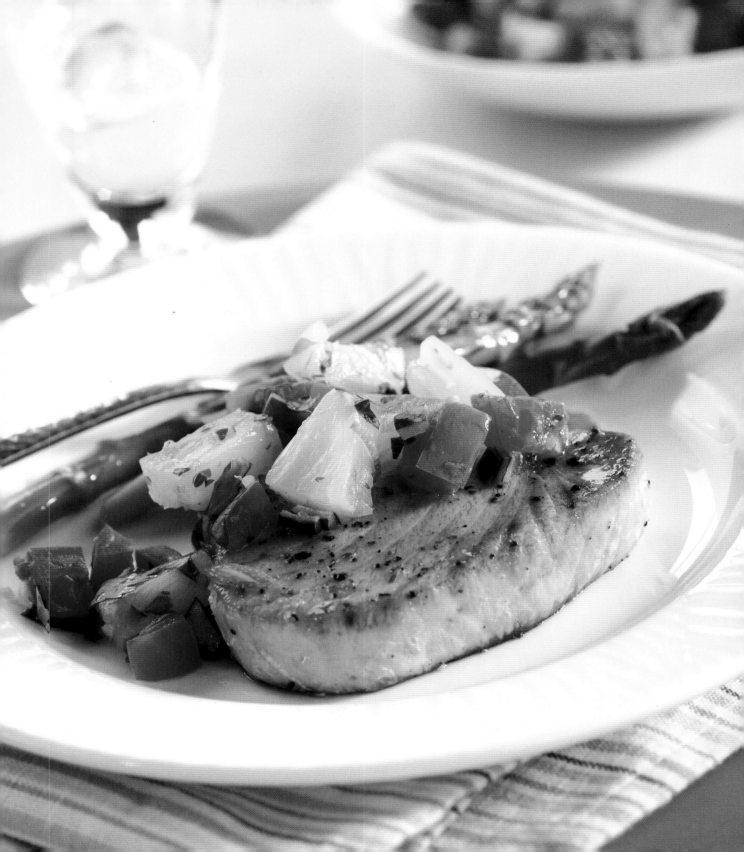

# BROILED HUNAN FISH FILLETS

Makes 4 servings

3 tablespoons coconut aminos

1 tablespoon finely chopped green onion

2 teaspoons dark sesame oil

1 clove garlic, minced

1 teaspoon minced fresh ginger

¼ teaspoon red pepper flakes

4 red snapper, scrod or cod fillets (5 to 7 ounces each)

**1.** Preheat broiler. Line broiler pan with foil.

**2.** Combine coconut aminos, green onion, oil, garlic, ginger and red pepper flakes in small bowl; mix well. Place fish on prepared pan; brush with garlic mixture.

**3.** Broil 4 to 5 inches from heat source 10 minutes or until fish begins to flake when tested with fork.

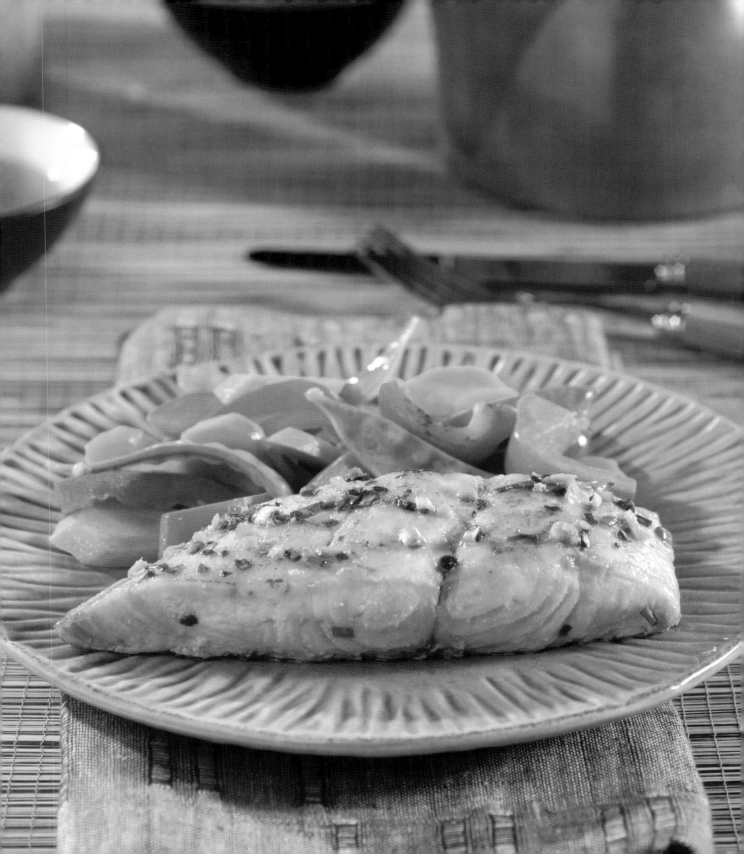

# SPICED SALMON WITH PINEAPPLE-GINGER SALSA

Makes 4 servings

1 tablespoon olive oil, plus additional for pan

4 salmon steaks (4 to 6 ounces each), rinsed and patted dry

1 teaspoon ground cumin

½ teaspoon ground allspice

½ teaspoon salt, divided

¼ teaspoon black pepper

¾ cup finely chopped fresh pineapple

¼ cup finely chopped poblano pepper

2 tablespoons chopped fresh cilantro

1 tablespoon lime juice

1 teaspoon grated fresh ginger

½ teaspoon grated orange peel

**1.** Preheat oven to 350°F. Line baking sheet with foil; brush lightly with oil. Place salmon on baking sheet.

**2.** Combine cumin, allspice, ¼ teaspoon salt and black pepper in small bowl; mix well. Brush salmon with 1 tablespoon oil; sprinkle both sides of fish with spice mixture.

**3.** Bake 14 to 16 minutes or until center is opaque.

**4.** Meanwhile, combine pineapple, poblano pepper, cilantro, lime juice, ginger, orange peel and remaining ¼ teaspoon salt in medium bowl; mix well. Serve salsa over fish.

**TIP:** Store fresh unpeeled ginger tightly wrapped in the refrigerator for up to 2 weeks.

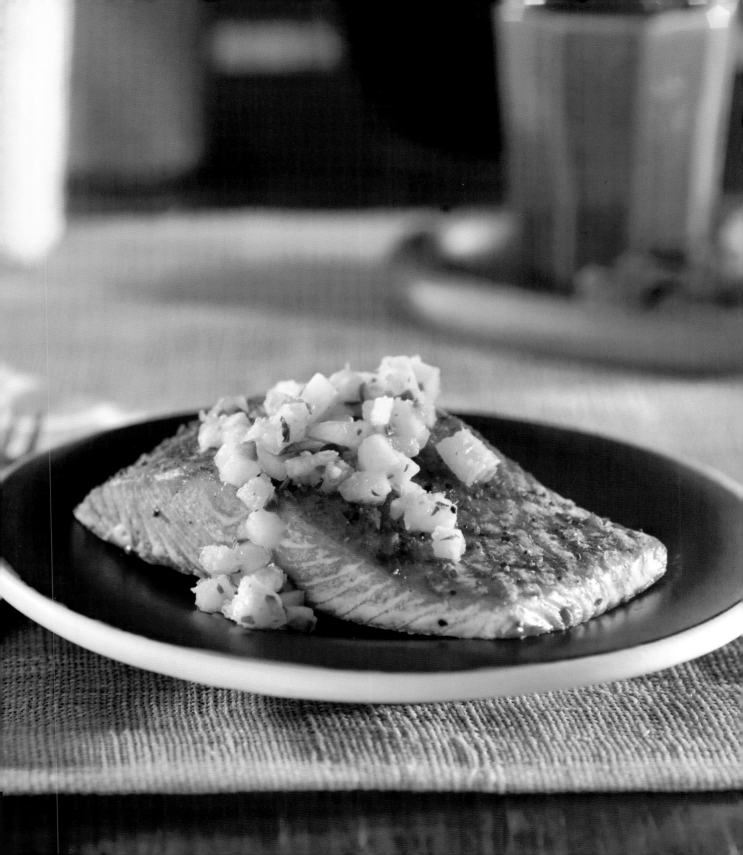

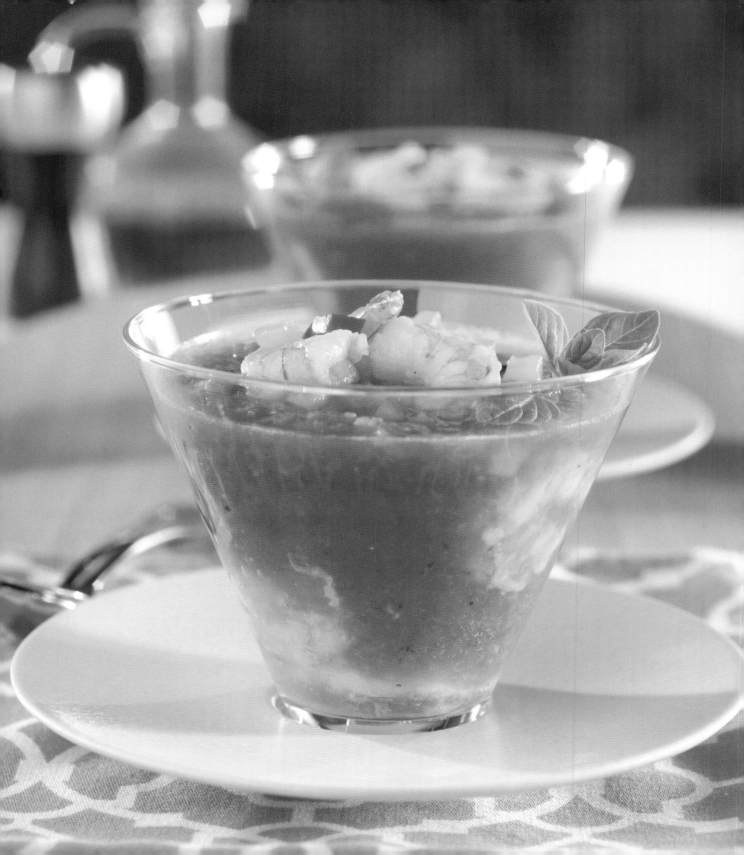

# SHELLFISH

## SHRIMP GAZPACHO

Makes 2 servings

1 tablespoon olive oil

8 ounces medium raw shrimp, peeled and deveined

½ teaspoon salt, divided

⅛ teaspoon black pepper

3 plum tomatoes, chopped (about 1½ cups)

¼ small red onion, chopped

¼ cucumber, peeled and chopped

¼ cup finely chopped roasted red and/or yellow peppers, divided

1 clove garlic, chopped

¾ cup tomato juice

1 tablespoon red wine vinegar

**1.** Heat oil in medium nonstick skillet over high heat. Season shrimp with ¼ teaspoon salt and black pepper. Add to skillet; cook 3 minutes or until shrimp are pink and opaque. Remove to plate.

**2.** Combine tomatoes, onion, cucumber, half of roasted peppers, garlic and remaining ¼ teaspoon salt in food processor; pulse until blended. Add tomato juice and vinegar; process until smooth.

**3.** Divide tomato mixture among glasses or bowls; top with shrimp and remaining roasted peppers.

# LEMON ROSEMARY SHRIMP AND VEGETABLE SOUVLAKI

### Makes 4 servings

3 tablespoons extra virgin olive oil, divided

2 tablespoons lemon juice

2 teaspoons grated lemon peel

2 cloves garlic, minced

½ teaspoon salt

½ teaspoon fresh rosemary leaves

⅛ teaspoon red pepper flakes

8 ounces large raw shrimp, peeled and deveined (with tails on)

1 medium zucchini, halved lengthwise and cut into ½-inch slices

½ medium red bell pepper, cut into 1-inch pieces

8 green onions, trimmed and cut into 2-inch pieces

**1.** Oil grid. Prepare grill for direct cooking. Soak four 12-inch wooden skewers in water 20 minutes to prevent burning.

**2.** Combine 2 tablespoons oil, lemon juice, lemon peel, garlic, salt, rosemary and red pepper flakes in small bowl; mix well.

**3.** Alternately thread shrimp, zucchini, bell pepper and green onions onto skewers. Brush with remaining 1 tablespoon oil.

**4.** Grill skewers over high heat 2 minutes per side or until shrimp are pink and opaque. Remove to serving platter; drizzle with sauce.

**NOTE:** "Souvlaki" is the Greek word for shishkebab. Souvlaki traditionally consists of fish or meat that has been seasoned in a mixture of oil, lemon juice, and seasonings. Many souvlaki recipes also include chunks of vegetables such as bell pepper and onion.

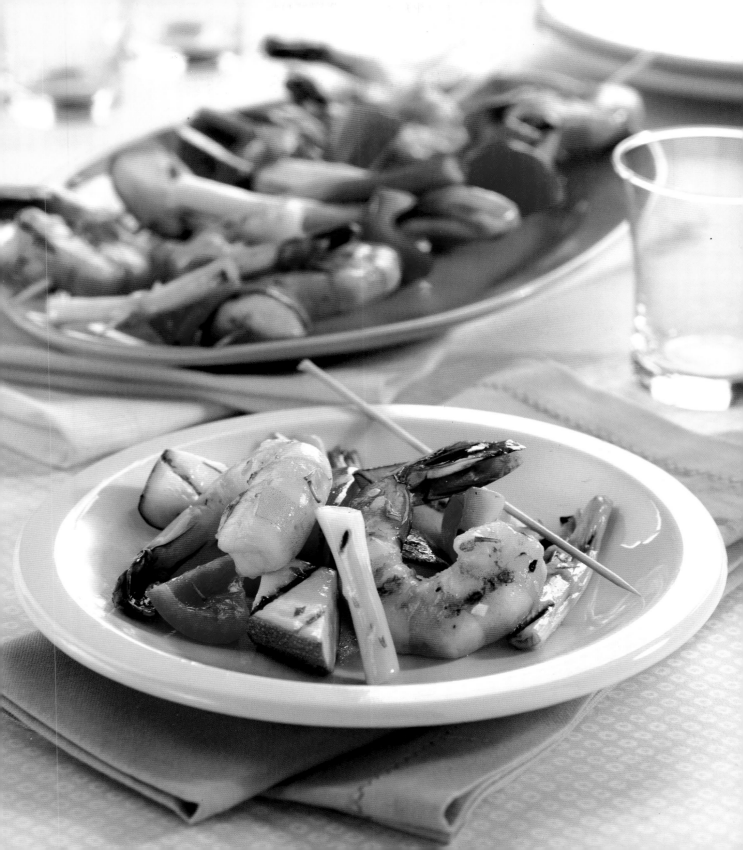

# BLACKENED SHRIMP WITH TOMATOES

Makes 4 servings

1½ teaspoons paprika

1 teaspoon Italian
  seasoning

½ teaspoon garlic
  powder

¼ teaspoon black
  pepper

8 ounces medium
  raw shrimp, peeled
  and deveined
  (with tails on)

1 tablespoon olive oil

1½ cups halved grape
  tomatoes

½ cup thinly sliced
  onion, separated
  into rings

  Lime wedges
  (optional)

**1.** Combine paprika, Italian seasoning, garlic powder and pepper in small bowl; mix well. Combine shrimp and spice mixture in large resealable food storage bag. Seal bag; shake to coat.

**2.** Heat oil in large skillet over medium-high heat. Add shrimp; cook 2 minutes per side or until shrimp are pink and opaque.

**3.** Add tomatoes and onion to skillet; cook 1 to 2 minutes or until tomatoes are heated through and onion is softened. Serve with lime wedges, if desired.

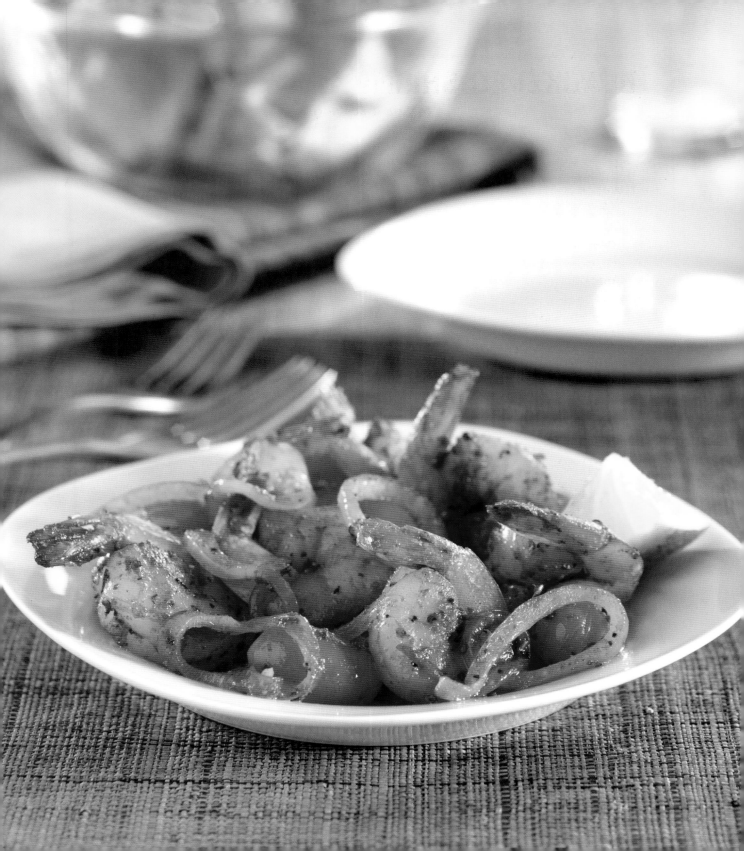

# GRILLED SCALLOPS AND VEGETABLES WITH CILANTRO SAUCE

Makes 4 servings

2 teaspoons dark sesame oil

¼ teaspoon red pepper flakes

1 green onion, chopped

1 tablespoon minced fresh ginger

1 cup chicken broth

1 cup chopped fresh cilantro

1 pound raw or thawed frozen sea scallops

2 medium zucchini, cut into ½-inch slices

2 medium yellow squash, cut into ½-inch slices

1 medium onion, cut into wedges

8 large mushrooms

**1.** Oil grid. Prepare grill for direct cooking.

**2.** Combine oil and red pepper flakes in small saucepan; heat over medium heat. Add green onion; cook about 15 seconds or just until fragrant. Add ginger; cook and stir 1 minute. Add broth; bring to a boil. Cook until liquid is reduced by half. Cool slightly.

**3.** Transfer mixture to blender or food processor. Add cilantro; blend until smooth.

**4.** Thread scallops and vegetables onto four 12-inch skewers. (If using wooden skewers, soak in water 20 minutes before using to prevent burning.)

**5.** Grill skewers over medium-high heat about 4 minutes per side or until scallops are opaque. Serve warm with cilantro sauce.

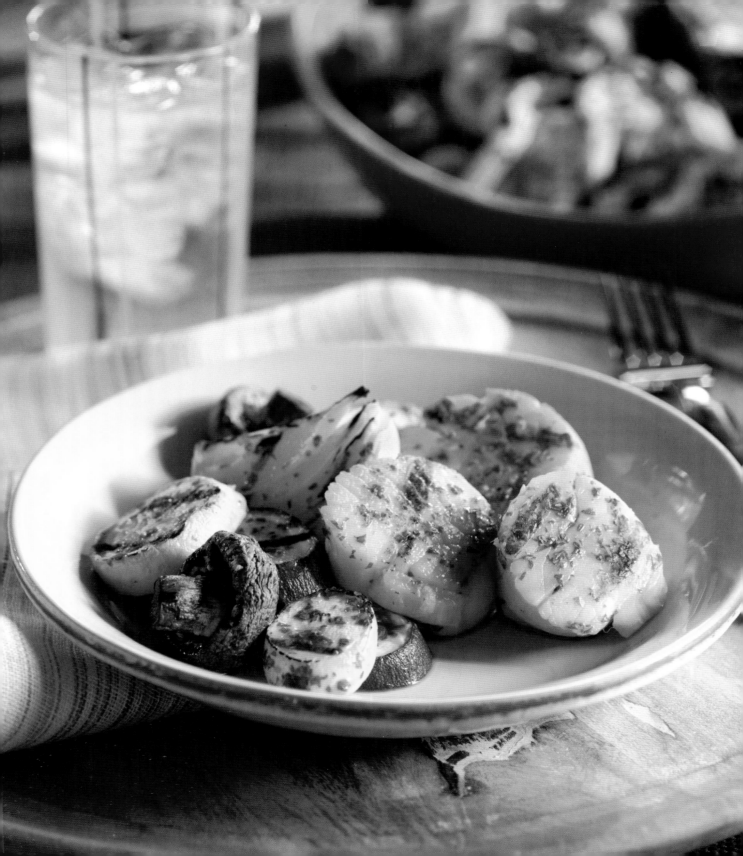

# SHRIMP AND TOMATO STIR-FRY

Makes 4 servings

20 kalamata olives,
   pitted and coarsely
   chopped

1 cup cherry tomatoes,
   halved

¼ cup chopped
   fresh basil

¼ teaspoon plus
   ⅛ teaspoon salt,
   divided

¼ teaspoon
   black pepper

2 tablespoons olive oil,
   divided

1 pound medium
   raw shrimp, peeled
   and deveined
   (with tails on)

1 clove garlic, minced

⅛ teaspoon red
   pepper flakes

1 medium zucchini,
   quartered
   lengthwise, then
   cut crosswise into
   2-inch pieces

1 medium onion, cut
   into 8 wedges

**1.** Combine olives, tomatoes, basil, ⅛ teaspoon salt and pepper in small bowl; mix well.

**2.** Heat 1 tablespoon oil in large nonstick skillet over medium heat. Add shrimp, garlic and red pepper flakes; cook and stir 3 minutes or until shrimp are pink and opaque. Remove to plate.

**3.** Add remaining 1 tablespoon oil to skillet; heat over medium-high heat. Add zucchini, onion and remaining ¼ teaspoon salt; cook and stir 5 minutes or until edges of vegetables begin to brown.

**4.** Add tomato mixture and shrimp to skillet; cook and stir 1 minute or until heated through.

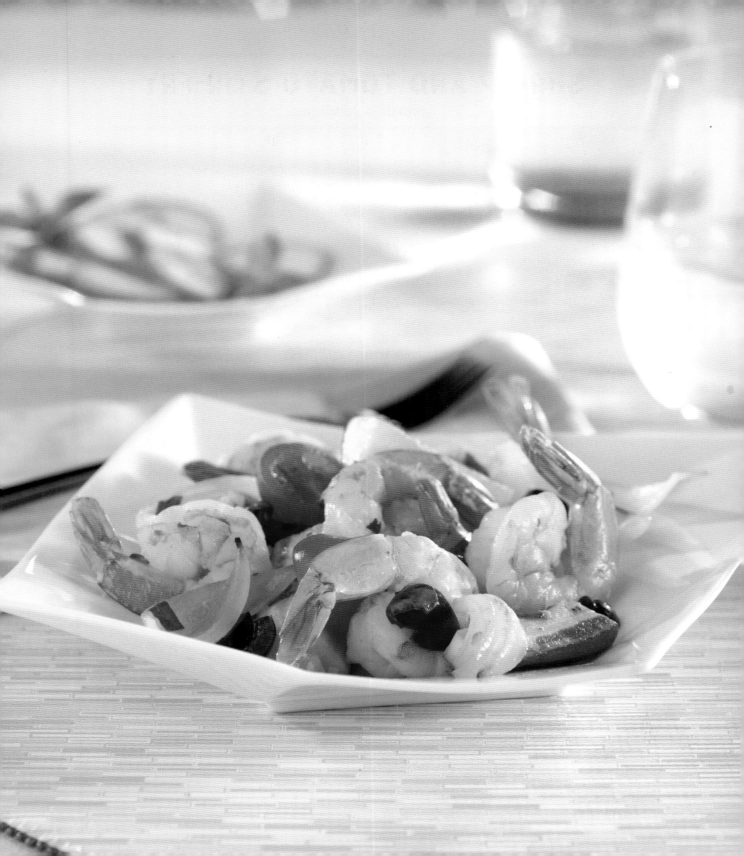

# SPICY THAI SHRIMP SOUP

## Makes 6 to 8 servings

1 tablespoon coconut oil

1 pound medium raw shrimp, peeled and deveined, shells reserved

1 jalapeño pepper,* cut into slivers

1 tablespoon paprika

¼ teaspoon ground red pepper

4 cans (about 14 ounces each) chicken broth

1 (½-inch) strip *each* lemon and lime peel

1 can (15 ounces) straw mushrooms, drained

Juice of 1 lemon

Juice of 1 lime

2 tablespoons coconut aminos

1 red Thai chile pepper or red jalapeño pepper,* cut into thin strips

¼ cup fresh cilantro leaves

*Chile peppers can sting and irritate the skin, so wear rubber gloves when handling peppers and do not touch your eyes.*

**1.** Heat large skillet over medium-high heat 1 minute. Add oil; heat 30 seconds. Add shrimp and jalapeño pepper; cook and stir 1 minute. Add paprika and ground red pepper; cook 1 minute or until shrimp are pink and opaque. Remove to medium bowl.

**2.** Add shrimp shells to skillet; cook and stir 30 seconds. Add broth and lemon and lime peels; bring to a boil. Reduce heat to low; cover and simmer 15 minutes.

**3.** Remove and discard shrimp shells and peels with slotted spoon. Add mushrooms and shrimp mixture to broth; bring to a boil over medium heat. Stir in lemon and lime juices, coconut aminos and Thai pepper; cook just until heated through. Sprinkle with cilantro.

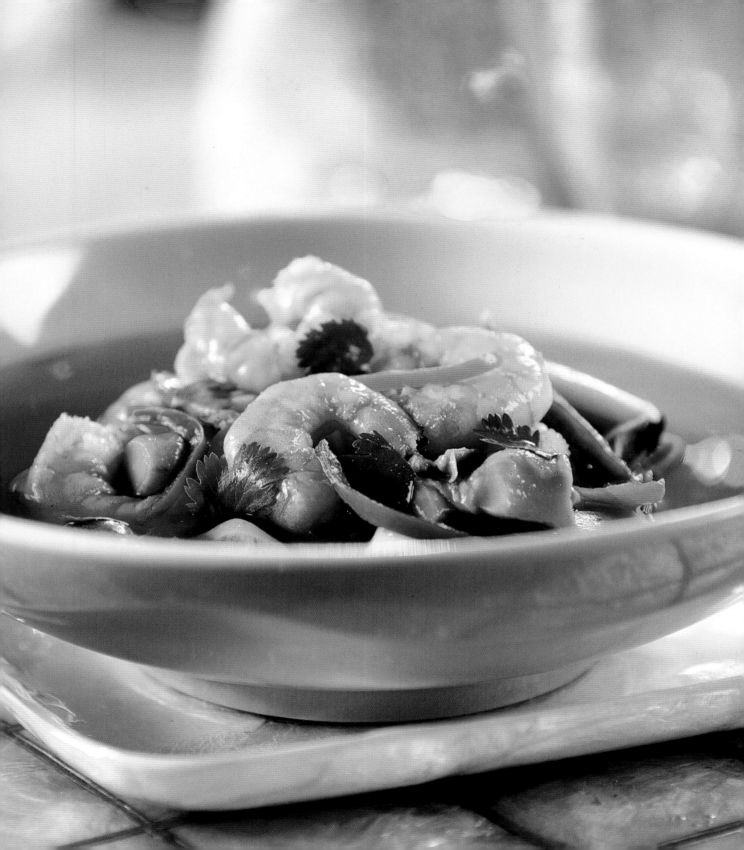

# CHICKEN AND SHRIMP JAMBALAYA

Makes 4 servings

- 1 package (about 12 ounces) riced cauliflower
- ¾ teaspoon salt
- ⅛ teaspoon black pepper
- ⅛ teaspoon ground red pepper
- 8 ounces boneless skinless chicken breast, cut into ½-inch pieces
- 1 tablespoon olive oil
- 1 onion, halved and cut into ¼-inch slices
- 1 *each* red, yellow and green bell pepper, cut into ¼-inch strips
- 2 cloves garlic, minced
- 1 large ripe tomato, chopped
- 8 ounces raw medium shrimp, peeled and deveined (with tails on)
- 1 cup chicken broth, divided
- 2 tablespoons chopped fresh parsley

**1.** Cook riced cauliflower according to package directions; set aside.

**2.** Combine salt, black pepper and ground red pepper in small bowl; mix well. Sprinkle half of mixture over chicken.

**3.** Heat oil in Dutch oven or large saucepan over medium heat. Add chicken; cook without stirring 2 minutes or until golden brown. Turn chicken; cook 2 minutes. Remove to plate.

**4.** Add onion and bell peppers to Dutch oven; cook and stir 3 minutes or until onion is translucent. Add garlic; cook and stir 1 minute. Stir in chicken, tomato, shrimp, ½ cup broth and remaining spice mixture; bring to a boil. Reduce heat to low; cook 5 minutes or until shrimp are pink and opaque.

**5.** Stir in riced cauliflower, remaining ½ cup broth and parsley; cook 3 minutes or until liquid is absorbed and cauliflower is heated through.

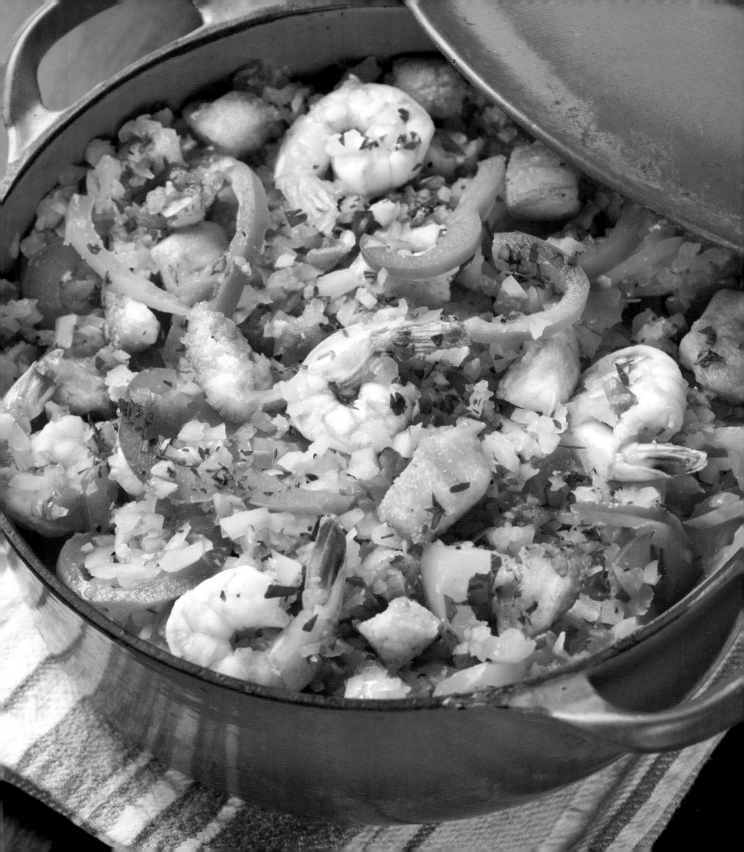

# CHIPOTLE SHRIMP AND SQUASH RIBBONS

Makes 4 servings

2   cloves garlic, peeled

1   canned chipotle pepper in adobo sauce, plus 1 teaspoon sauce

2   tablespoons water

¼   teaspoon salt

2   medium zucchini

2   medium yellow squash

1   tablespoon olive oil

1   small onion, diced

1   medium red bell pepper, cut into strips

8   ounces medium raw shrimp, peeled and deveined

    Lime wedges (optional)

**1.** Combine garlic, chipotle pepper with adobo sauce, water and salt in food processor; process until smooth.

**2.** Shave zucchini and yellow squash into ribbons with vegetable peeler. (Discard seedy centers.)

**3.** Heat oil in large skillet over high heat. Add onion and bell pepper; cook and stir 1 minute. Add shrimp and chipotle mixture; cook and stir 2 minutes. Add zucchini and yellow squash; cook and stir 1 to 2 minutes or until squash are slightly wilted and shrimp are pink and opaque. Serve with lime wedges, if desired.

**NOTE:** Chipotle peppers are smoked jalapeños. They're usually found canned with adobo sauce, which is a dark red sauce made of chili peppers, herbs and vinegar. Leftover chipotle peppers with adobo sauce can be frozen in resealable freezer food storage bags or in an airtight container.

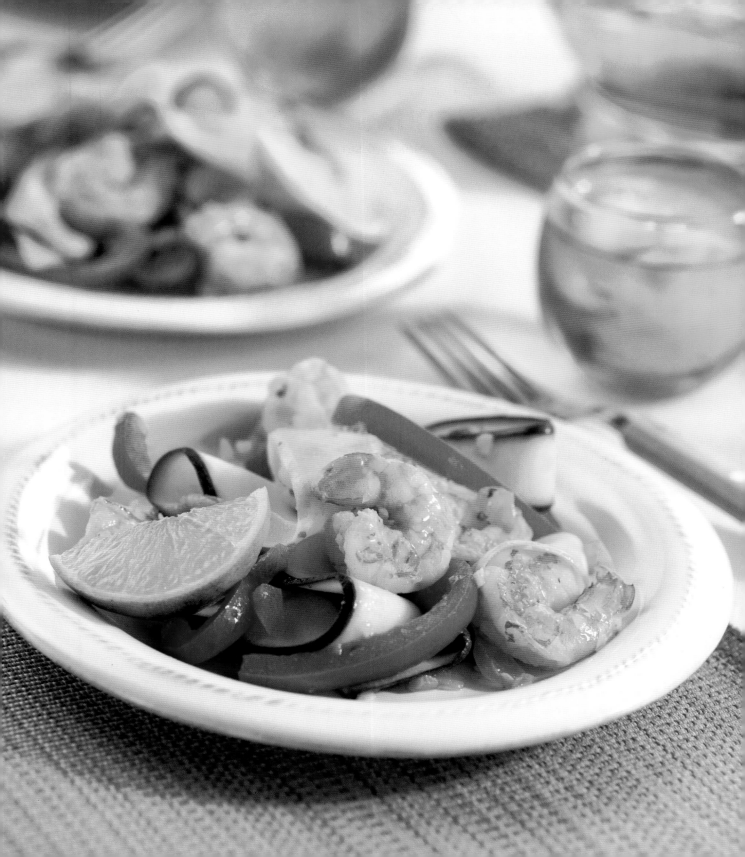

# SAVORY SEAFOOD SOUP

Makes 4 servings

2½ cups water

1½ cups dry white wine

1 onion, chopped

½ red bell pepper, chopped

½ green bell pepper, chopped

1 clove garlic, minced

½ teaspoon salt

8 ounces halibut, cut into 1-inch pieces

8 ounces sea scallops, cut into halves

1 teaspoon dried thyme

Juice of ½ lime

Dash hot pepper sauce

Black pepper

**1.** Combine water, wine, onion, bell peppers, garlic and ½ teaspoon salt in large saucepan; bring to a boil over high heat. Reduce heat to medium-low; cover and simmer 15 minutes or until bell peppers are tender, stirring occasionally.

**2.** Add halibut, scallops and thyme; cook 2 minutes or until fish and scallops are opaque. Stir in lime juice and hot pepper sauce. Season with additional salt and black pepper.

**TIP:** If halibut is not available, cod, ocean perch or haddock can be substituted.

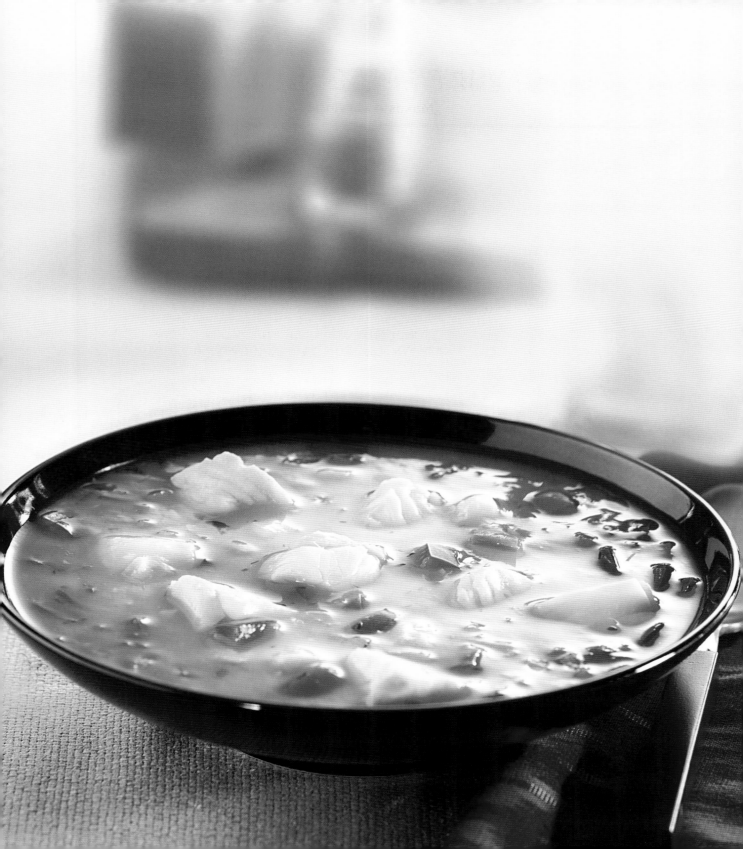

# SHRIMP AND VEGGIE SKILLET TOSS

Makes 4 servings

¼ cup coconut aminos

2 tablespoons lime juice

1 tablespoon dark sesame oil

1 teaspoon grated fresh ginger

⅛ teaspoon red pepper flakes

1 tablespoon olive oil, divided

8 ounces medium raw shrimp, peeled and deveined (with tails on)

2 medium zucchini, cut in half lengthwise and thinly sliced

6 green onions, trimmed and halved lengthwise

16 grape tomatoes

1. Combine coconut aminos, lime juice, sesame oil, ginger and red pepper flakes in small bowl; mix well.

2. Heat half of olive oil in large nonstick skillet over medium-high heat. Add shrimp; cook and stir 3 minutes or until pink and opaque. Remove to large bowl.

3. Heat remaining olive oil in skillet. Add zucchini; cook and stir 4 to 6 minutes or until crisp-tender. Add green onions and tomatoes; cook and stir 2 minutes. Add shrimp, cook 1 minute or until heated through. Return shrimp and vegetables to large bowl.

4. Add sauce mixture to skillet; bring to a boil. Remove from heat. Stir in shrimp and vegetables; toss gently to coat.

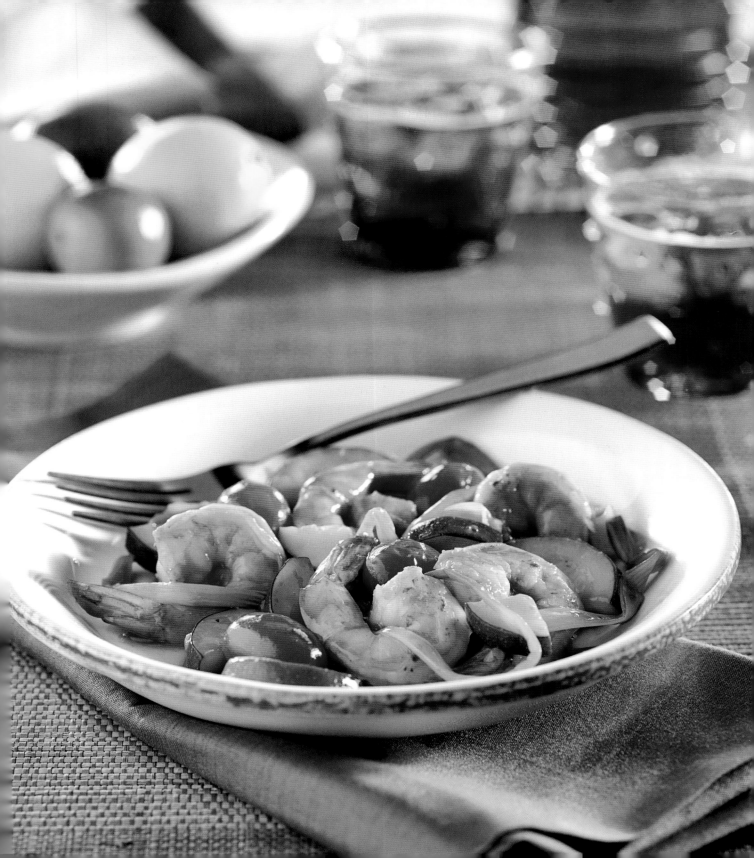

# SEARED SCALLOPS OVER GARLIC-LEMON SPINACH

Makes 4 servings

1 pound sea scallops (about 12)

1 tablespoon olive oil

¼ teaspoon salt

⅛ teaspoon black pepper

2 cloves garlic, minced

1 shallot, minced

1 package (about 6 ounces) baby spinach

1 tablespoon lemon juice

Lemon wedges (optional)

**1.** Pat scallops dry with paper towels. Heat oil in large nonstick skillet over medium-high heat. Add scallops; sprinkle with salt and pepper. Cook 2 to 3 minutes per side or until golden brown and opaque. Remove to plate; tent with foil.

**2.** Add garlic and shallot to skillet; cook and stir 45 seconds or until fragrant. Add spinach; cook 2 minutes or just until spinach begins to wilt, stirring occasionally. Remove from heat; stir in lemon juice.

**3.** Serve scallops over spinach. Garnish with lemon wedges.

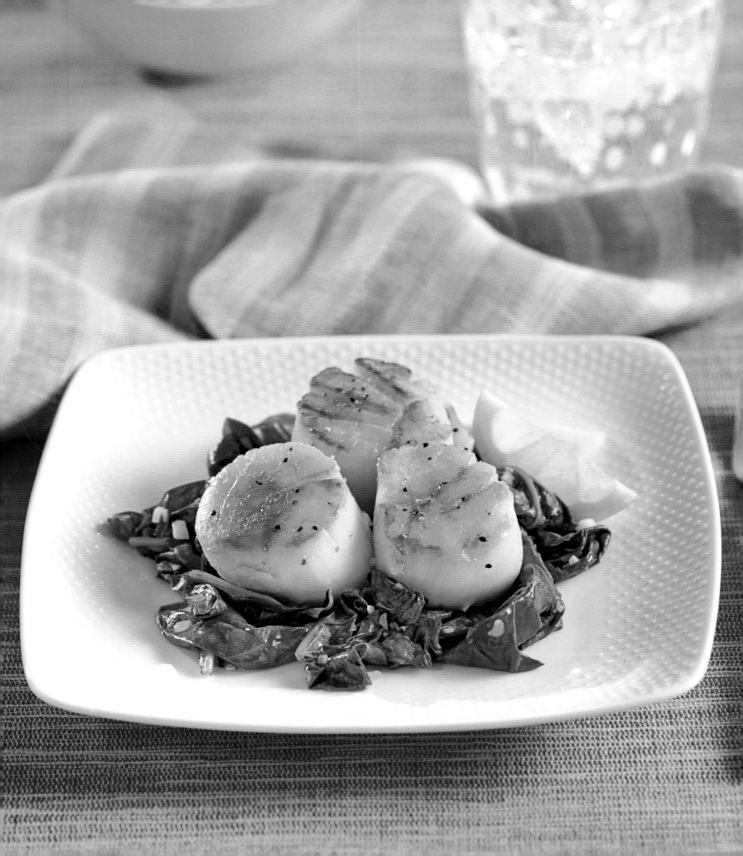

# GAZPACHO SHRIMP SALAD

Makes 4 servings

½ cup chunky salsa

1 tablespoon olive oil

1 tablespoon balsamic vinegar

1 clove garlic, minced

8 cups torn mixed salad greens or romaine lettuce

1 large tomato, chopped

1 small ripe avocado, diced

½ cup thinly sliced unpeeled cucumber

½ pound large cooked shrimp, peeled and deveined

½ cup coarsely chopped fresh cilantro

**1.** Combine salsa, oil, vinegar and garlic in small bowl; mix well.

**2.** Combine greens, tomato, avocado and cucumber in large bowl. Divide salad among four plates; top with shrimp.

**3.** Drizzle dressing over salads; sprinkle with cilantro.

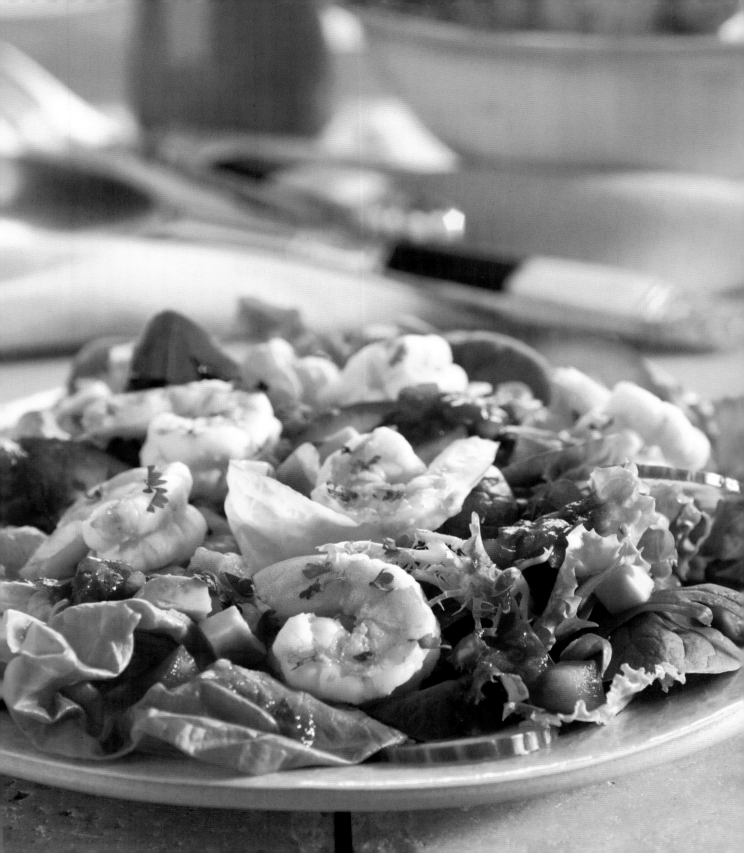

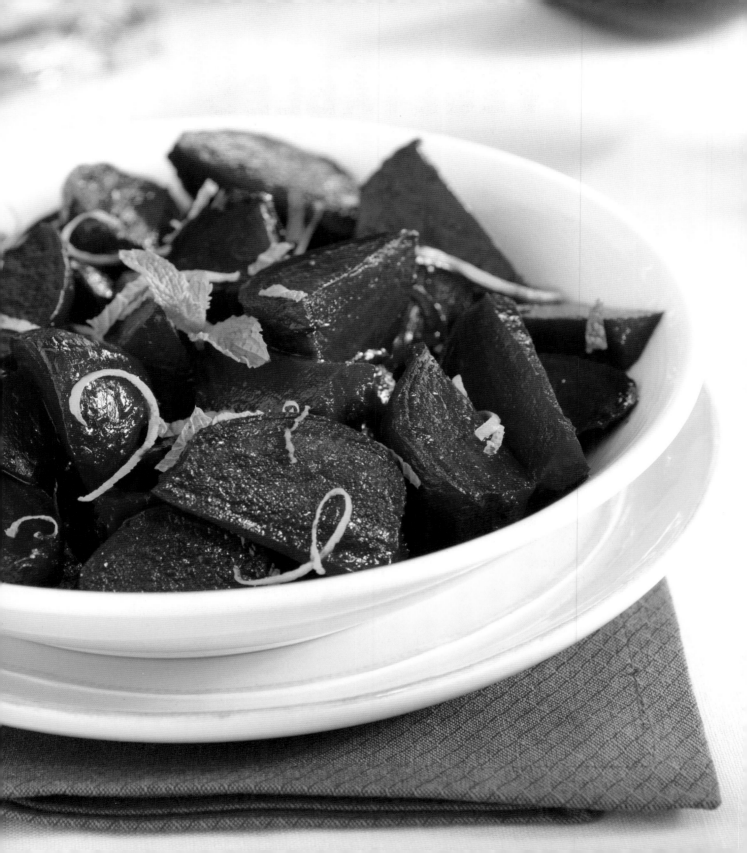

# VEGETABLES

## ORANGE AND MAPLE GLAZED ROASTED BEETS

Makes 4 servings

4 medium beets, scrubbed

1 tablespoon olive oil

¼ cup orange juice

3 tablespoons balsamic or cider vinegar

2 tablespoons maple syrup

2 teaspoons grated orange peel, divided

1 teaspoon Dijon mustard

1 to 2 tablespoons chopped fresh mint (optional)

Salt and black pepper

**1.** Preheat oven to 425°F. Place beets in glass baking dish. Drizzle with oil; toss to coat.

**2.** Cover and roast 45 minutes to 1 hour or until small knife inserted into largest beet goes in easily. Let stand until cool enough to handle.

**3.** Peel and cut beets in half lengthwise; cut into wedges. Return to baking dish.

**4.** Whisk orange juice, vinegar, maple syrup, 1 teaspoon orange peel and mustard in small bowl until well blended. Pour over beets; mix gently.

**5.** Roast 10 to 15 minutes or until heated through and liquid is absorbed. Sprinkle with remaining 1 teaspoon orange peel and mint, if desired. Season with salt and pepper.

# KALE WITH LEMON AND GARLIC

Makes 6 to 8 servings

2 bunches kale
   or Swiss chard
   (1 to 1¼ pounds)

1 tablespoon olive oil

3 cloves garlic, minced

½ cup chicken or
   vegetable broth

½ teaspoon salt

¼ teaspoon
   black pepper

1 lemon, cut into
   wedges

**1.** Trim tough stems from kale. Stack and thinly slice leaves.

**2.** Heat oil in large saucepan over medium heat. Add garlic; cook 3 minutes, stirring occasionally. Add kale and broth; cover and cook 7 minutes. Stir kale; cover and cook over medium-low heat 8 to 10 minutes or until kale is tender.

**3.** Stir in salt and pepper. Squeeze wedge of lemon over each serving.

# BUTTERNUT SQUASH OVEN FRIES

Makes 4 servings

½ teaspoon salt

½ teaspoon
   garlic powder

¼ teaspoon ground
   red pepper

1 butternut squash
   (about 2½ pounds),
   peeled, seeded and
   cut into 2-inch-thin
   strips

1 tablespoon
   coconut oil

**1.** Preheat oven to 425°F. Combine salt, garlic powder and red pepper in small bowl; mix well.

**2.** Place squash on baking sheet. Drizzle with oil and sprinkle with seasoning mixture; toss gently to coat. Spread in single layer.

**3.** Bake 20 to 25 minutes or until squash just begins to brown, stirring occasionally. *Turn oven to broil.*

**4.** Broil 3 to 5 minutes or until squash is browned and crisp. Spread on paper towels to cool slightly before serving.

Kale with Lemon
and Garlic

# SPICY RATATOUILLE WITH SPAGHETTI SQUASH

Makes 4 servings

1 spaghetti squash
(about 2 pounds)

2 tablespoons olive oil

1 small onion,
finely chopped

1 clove garlic, minced

1 small eggplant, diced

1 small zucchini, diced

1 cup coarsely chopped
mushrooms,
preferably oyster
or shiitake

1 can (about 14 ounces)
diced tomatoes

1 tablespoon canned
chipotle pepper
in adobo sauce,
minced

¾ teaspoon salt

½ teaspoon
dried oregano

¼ teaspoon
black pepper

**1.** Pierce squash skin with fork or paring knife several times; place in microwavable dish. Cover loosely with plastic wrap; microwave on HIGH 12 to 13 minutes, turning squash over after 6 minutes. (Squash is fully cooked when fork pierces skin and flesh easily.) Set squash aside until cool enough to handle.

**2.** Cut squash in half lengthwise. If necessary, use towel to hold warm squash; scoop out and discard seeds. Rake fork across flesh, against the grain, to separate squash into strands. Measure 2 cups squash; cover and set aside. Reserve empty squash shell halves for serving, if desired.

**3.** While squash cooks, heat oil in large skillet over medium-high heat. Add onion and garlic; cook and stir 1 minute. Add eggplant, zucchini and mushrooms; cook 5 minutes or until vegetables are lightly browned, stirring occasionally. Stir in tomatoes, chipotle pepper, salt, oregano and black pepper; cook over medium heat 5 minutes or until slightly thickened and heated through.

**4.** Spread squash strands in serving bowl or in reserved squash shells; top with ratatouille. Serve immediately.

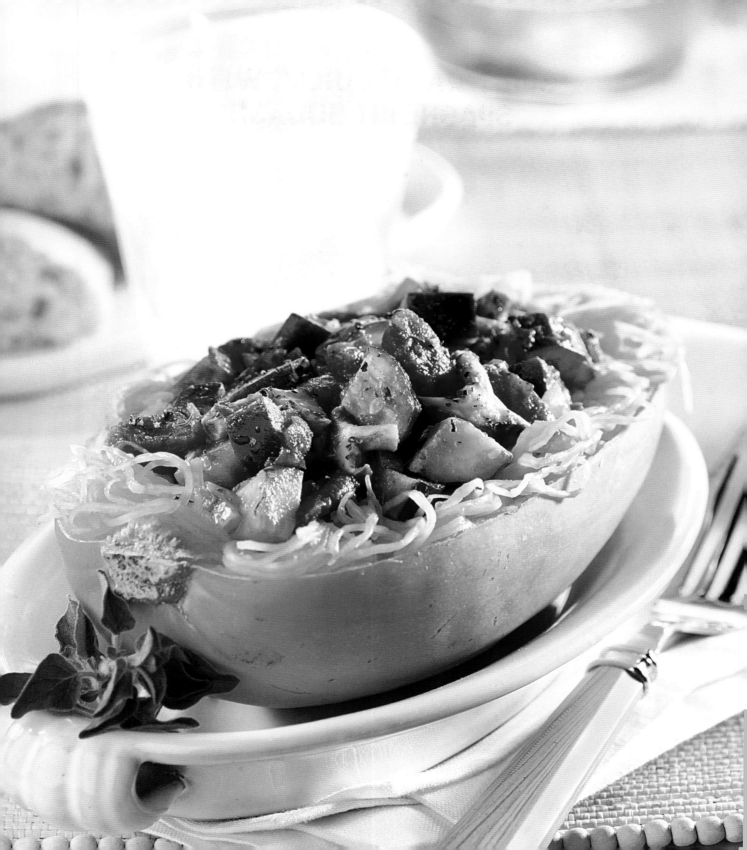

# ASPARAGUS WITH RED ONION, BASIL AND ALMONDS

## Makes 4 servings

2 tablespoons butter

½ cup thinly sliced red onion, separated into rings

1 pound asparagus, trimmed and cut into 1½-inch pieces

¼ cup chicken or vegetable broth

2 tablespoons chopped fresh basil

½ teaspoon salt

¼ teaspoon black pepper

2 tablespoons sliced almonds, toasted*

*To toast almonds, cook in small skillet over medium-low heat about 5 minutes or until lightly browned, stirring frequently.*

**1.** Melt butter in small skillet over medium heat. Add onion; cover and cook 5 minutes or until tender. Uncover; cook 5 minutes or until golden brown, stirring occasionally.

**2.** Combine asparagus and broth in medium saucepan; cover and bring to a boil over high heat. Reduce heat to low; cook 4 minutes.

**3.** Stir in onion; cook, uncovered, about 2 minutes or until asparagus is crisp-tender and most liquid is evaporated. Stir in basil, salt and pepper. Sprinkle with almonds.

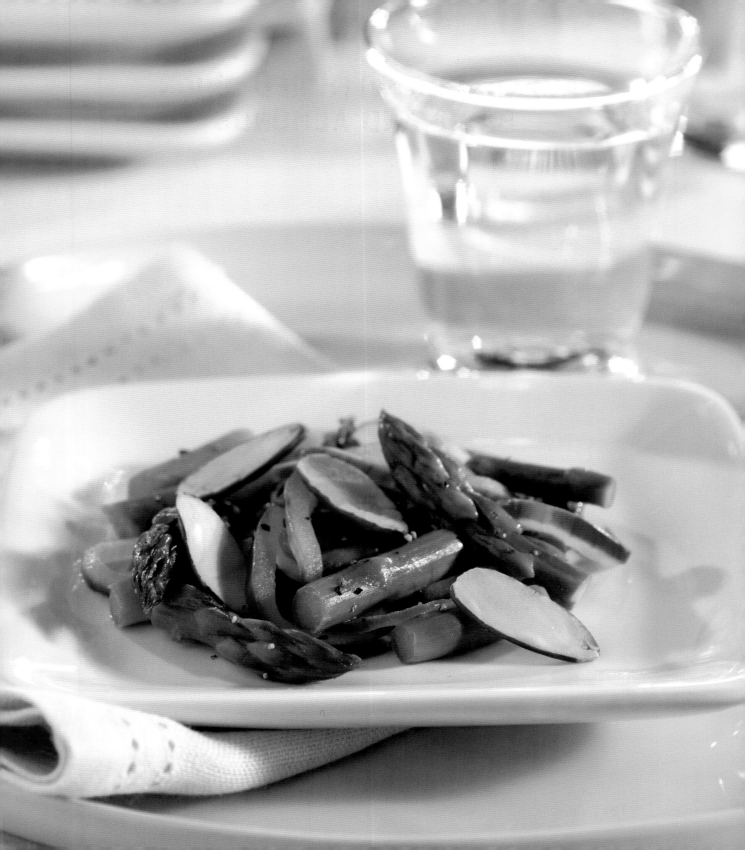

# ROASTED CREMINI MUSHROOMS

Makes 4 servings

1 pound cremini
   mushrooms, halved

½ cup sliced shallots

1 tablespoon olive oil

½ teaspoon coarse salt

½ teaspoon dried
   rosemary

¼ teaspoon black pepper

Fresh rosemary
(optional)

**1.** Preheat oven to 400°F.

**2.** Combine mushrooms and shallots on baking sheet. Combine oil, salt, dried rosemary and pepper in small bowl; mix well. Pour over mushrooms and shallots; toss to coat. Spread vegetables in single layer on baking sheet.

**3.** Roast 15 to 18 minutes or until mushrooms are browned and tender. Garnish with fresh rosemary.

# MIDDLE EASTERN SPINACH SALAD

Makes 4 servings

¼ cup lemon juice

1 tablespoon olive oil

2 teaspoons honey

½ teaspoon salt

½ teaspoon curry powder

1 pound fresh spinach,
   stemmed and patted
   dry

½ cup golden raisins

¼ cup minced red onion

¼ cup thin red onion
   slices

**1.** Whisk lemon juice, oil, honey, salt and curry powder in small bowl until well blended.

**2.** Tear spinach into bite-size pieces. Combine spinach, raisins, minced onion and onion slices in large bowl. Add dressing; toss gently to coat.

Roasted Cremini
Mushrooms

# GLAZED PARSNIPS AND CARROTS

### Makes 6 servings

1 pound parsnips
(2 large or
3 medium)

1 package (8 ounces)
baby carrots

1 tablespoon olive oil

Salt and black pepper

¼ cup orange juice

1 tablespoon butter

1 tablespoon honey

¼ teaspoon salt

⅛ teaspoon ground
ginger

**1.** Preheat oven to 425°F. Peel parsnips; cut into sticks to match size of baby carrots.

**2.** Combine vegetables on baking sheet. Drizzle with oil and season with salt and pepper; toss to coat. Spread in single layer. Bake 30 to 35 minutes or until fork-tender.

**3.** Combine orange juice, butter, honey, salt and ginger in large skillet; mix well. Add vegetables; cook and stir over high heat 1 to 2 minutes or until glazed.

# BROCCOLI ITALIAN STYLE

### Makes 4 servings

1¼ pounds fresh broccoli

2 tablespoons lemon
juice

1 tablespoon extra
virgin olive oil

1 clove garlic, minced

1 teaspoon chopped
fresh Italian parsley

½ teaspoon salt

Dash black pepper

**1.** Trim broccoli, discarding tough stems. Cut broccoli into florets with 2-inch stems. Peel remaining stems; cut into ½-inch slices.

**2.** Bring 1 quart water to a boil in large saucepan over medium-high heat. Add broccoli; return to a boil. Cook 3 to 5 minutes or until broccoli is tender. Drain and transfer to serving dish.

**3.** Combine lemon juice, oil, garlic, parsley, salt and pepper in small bowl; mix well. Pour over broccoli; toss to coat. Cover and let stand 1 hour before serving to allow flavors to blend. Serve at room temperature.

Glazed Parsnips
and Carrots

# MARKET SALAD

Makes 4 servings

3 eggs

4 cups mixed baby
  salad greens

2 cups green beans, cut
  into 1½-inch pieces,
  cooked and drained

4 slices thick-cut
  bacon, crisp-cooked
  and crumbled

1 tablespoon minced
  fresh basil, chives
  or Italian parsley

3 tablespoons extra
  virgin olive oil

1 tablespoon red
  wine vinegar

1 teaspoon
  Dijon mustard

¼ teaspoon salt

¼ teaspoon
  black pepper

**1.** Place eggs in small saucepan; add enough water to cover. Bring to a boil over medium-high heat. Immediately remove from heat; cover and let stand 10 minutes. Drain eggs; cool to room temperature.

**2.** Combine salad greens, green beans, bacon and basil in large serving bowl. Peel and coarsely chop eggs; add to bowl.

**3.** Combine oil, vinegar, mustard, salt and pepper in small bowl; mix well. Drizzle dressing over salad; toss gently to coat.

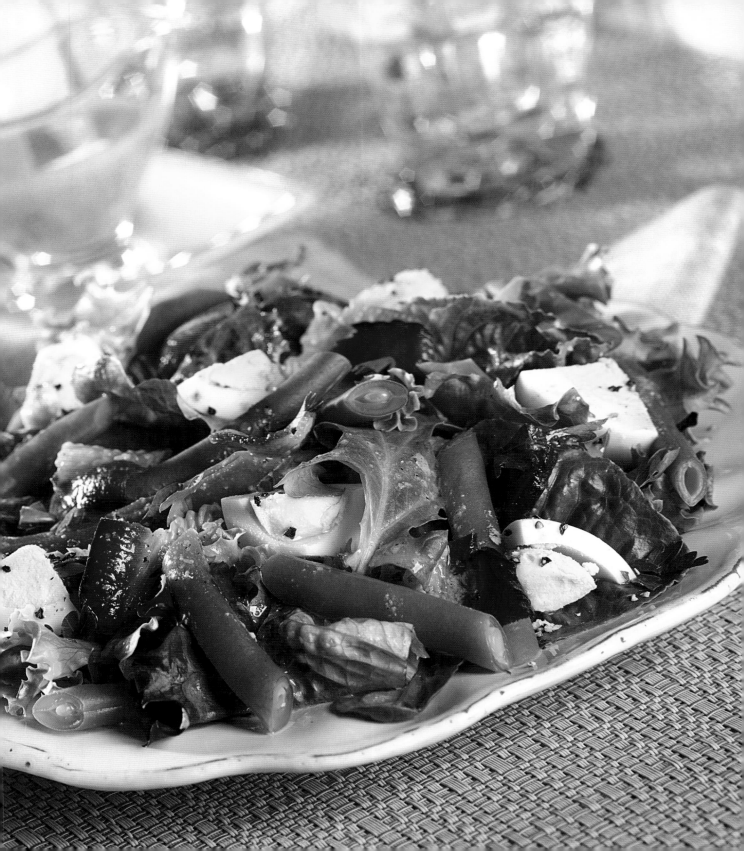

# TANGY RED CABBAGE
# WITH APPLES AND BACON

Makes 4 servings

8 slices thick-cut bacon

1 large onion, sliced

½ small head red
   cabbage (1 pound),
   thinly sliced

2 teaspoons honey

1 Granny Smith apple,
   peeled and sliced

2 tablespoons
   cider vinegar

½ teaspoon salt

¼ teaspoon
   black pepper

**1.** Cook bacon in large skillet over medium-high heat 6 to 8 minutes or until crisp, turning occasionally. Drain on paper towel-lined plate. Coarsely chop bacon.

**2.** Drain all but 2 tablespoons drippings from skillet. Add onion to skillet; cook and stir over medium-high heat 2 to 3 minutes or until onion begins to soften. Add cabbage and honey; cook and stir 4 to 5 minutes or until cabbage wilts.

**3.** Stir in apple; cook 3 minutes or until crisp-tender. Stir in vinegar; cook 1 minute or until absorbed.

**4.** Stir in bacon, salt and pepper; cook 1 minute or until heated through. Serve warm or at room temperature.

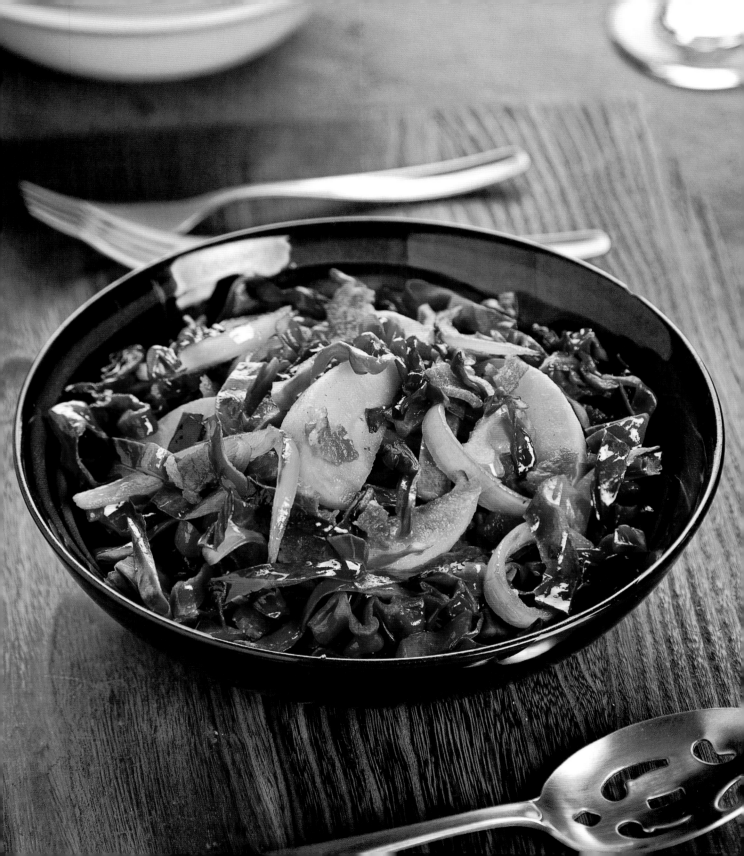

# SWEET AND SAVORY SWEET POTATO SALAD

Makes 6 servings

4 cups peeled chopped cooked sweet potatoes (4 to 6)

¾ cup chopped green onions

½ cup chopped fresh parsley

½ cup unsweetened dried cherries

¼ cup plus 2 tablespoons rice wine vinegar

2 tablespoons extra virgin olive oil

2 tablespoons coarse ground mustard

¾ teaspoon garlic powder

½ teaspoon salt

¼ teaspoon black pepper

1. Combine sweet potatoes, green onions, parsley and cherries in large bowl.

2. Whisk vinegar, oil, mustard, garlic powder, salt and pepper in small bowl until well blended.

3. Pour dressing over salad; toss gently to coat. Serve immediately or cover and refrigerate until ready to serve.

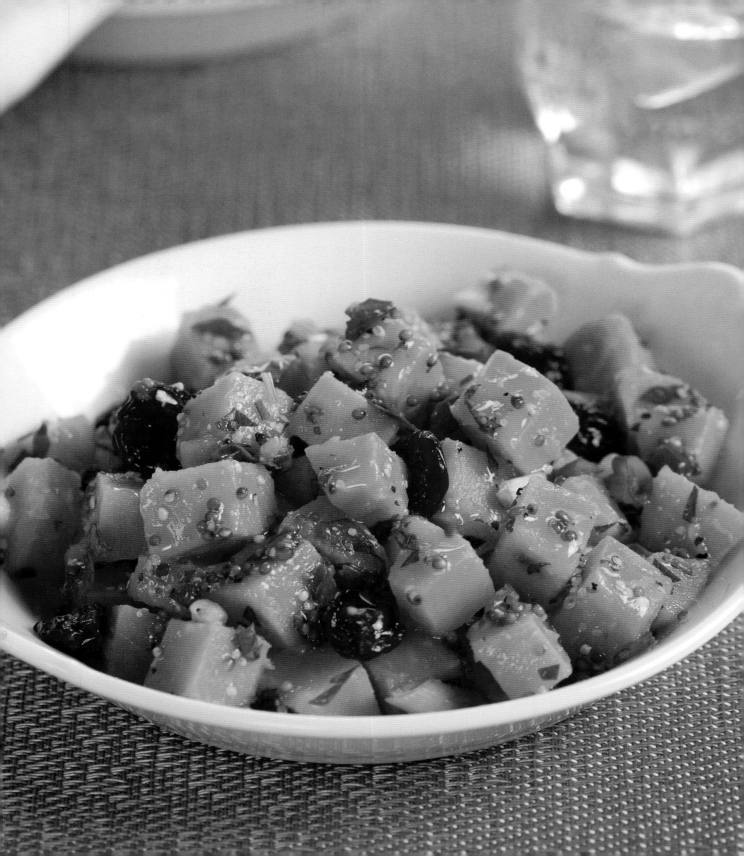

# MEDITERRANEAN VEGETABLE BAKE

Makes 4 to 6 servings

3 tablespoons olive oil, plus additional for baking dish

1 small red onion

1 medium zucchini

1 small yellow squash

2 tomatoes, sliced

1 small eggplant, sliced

1 large portobello mushroom, sliced

2 cloves garlic, finely chopped

2 teaspoons chopped fresh rosemary leaves

⅔ cup dry white wine

Salt and black pepper

**1.** Preheat oven to 350°F. Brush 13×9-inch baking dish or shallow casserole with oil.

**2.** Spiral red onion, zucchini and yellow squash with thick spiral blade.* Layer spiraled vegetables, tomatoes, eggplant and mushroom alternately in prepared baking dish. Sprinkle evenly with garlic.

**3.** Combine 3 tablespoons oil and rosemary in small bowl; drizzle over vegetables. Pour wine over vegetables; season with salt and pepper. Cover loosely with foil.

**4.** Bake 20 minutes. Uncover; bake 10 to 15 minutes or until vegetables are tender.

*If you don't have a spiralizer, cut onion, zucchini and yellow squash into thin strips.*

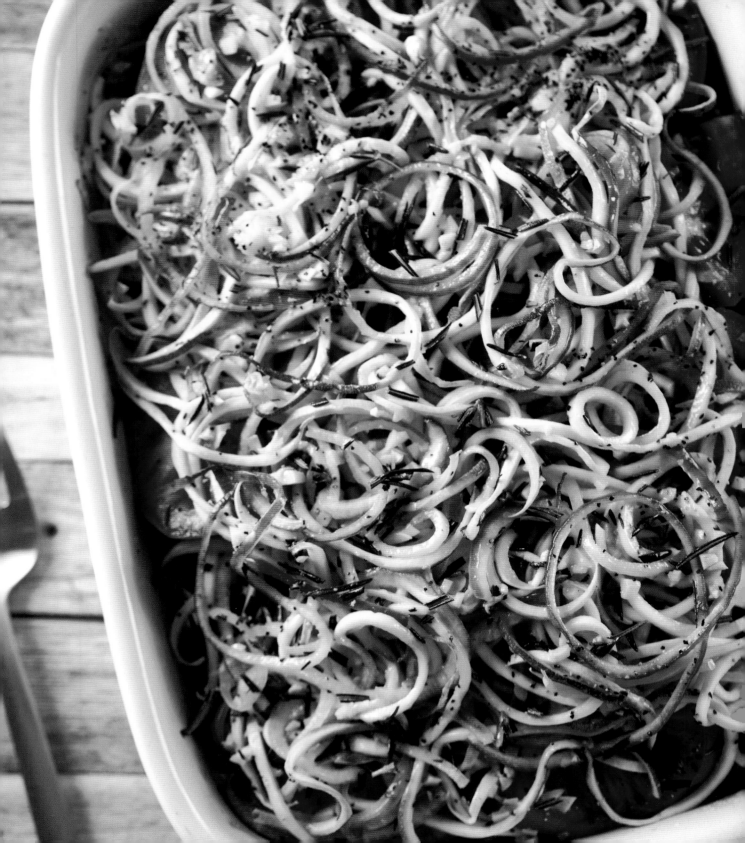

# ROASTED CURRIED CAULIFLOWER AND BRUSSELS SPROUTS

Makes 10 servings

2 pounds cauliflower florets

12 ounces brussels sprouts, trimmed and cut in half lengthwise

⅓ cup olive oil

2½ tablespoons curry powder

½ teaspoon salt

½ teaspoon black pepper

½ cup chopped fresh cilantro

**1.** Preheat oven to 400°F. Line large baking sheet with foil.

**2.** Combine cauliflower, brussels sprouts and oil in large bowl; toss to coat. Sprinkle with curry powder, salt and pepper; toss again. Spread vegetables in single layer on prepared baking sheet.

**3.** Roast 25 to 30 minutes or until golden brown, stirring after 15 minutes. Stir in cilantro.

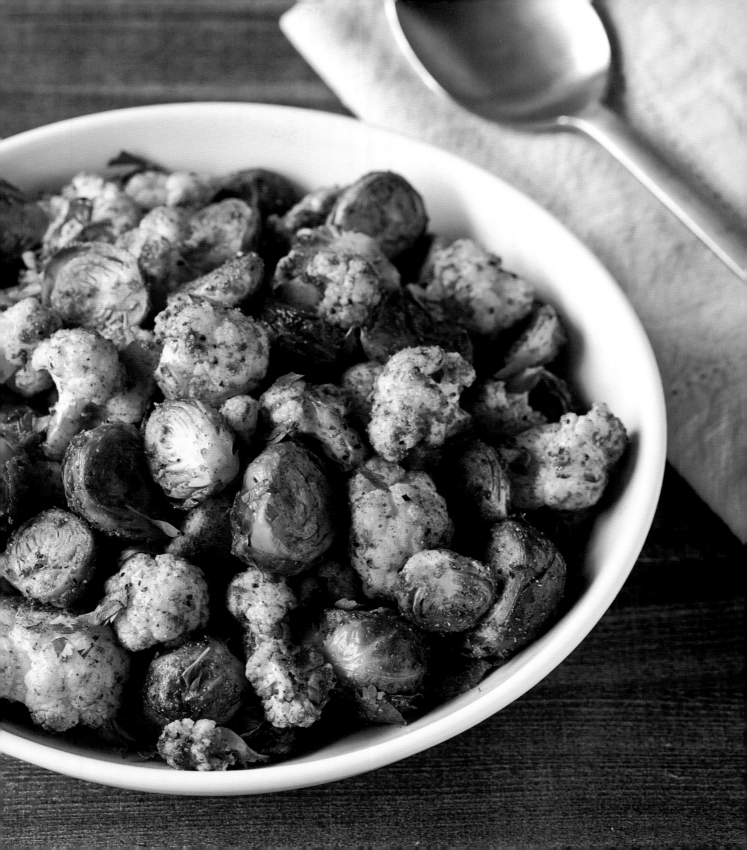

# BALSAMIC BUTTERNUT SQUASH

Makes 4 servings

3 tablespoons olive oil

2 tablespoons thinly sliced fresh sage (about 6 large leaves), divided

1 medium butternut squash, peeled and cut into 1-inch pieces (4 to 5 cups)

½ red onion, cut in half then cut into ¼-inch slices

1 teaspoon salt, divided

2½ tablespoons balsamic vinegar

¼ teaspoon black pepper

**1.** Heat oil in large cast iron skillet over medium-high heat. Add 1 tablespoon sage; cook and stir 3 minutes. Add squash, onion and ½ teaspoon salt; cook 6 minutes, stirring occasionally. Reduce heat to medium; cook 15 minutes without stirring.

**2.** Stir in vinegar, remaining ½ teaspoon salt and pepper; cook 10 minutes or until squash is tender, stirring occasionally. Stir in remaining 1 tablespoon sage; cook 1 minute.

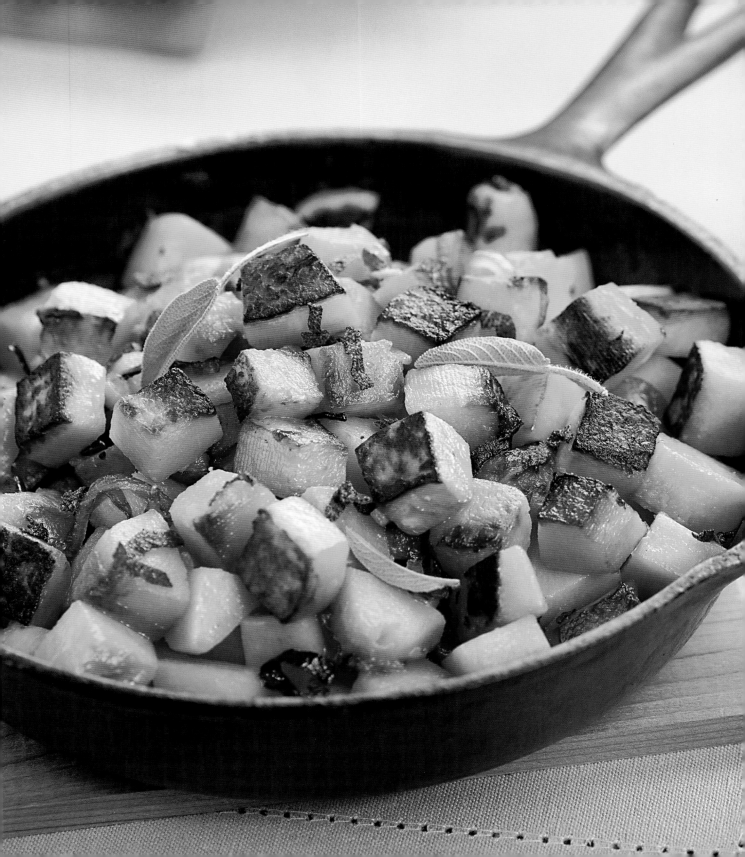

# SPINACH-MELON SALAD

Makes 6 servings

6 cups packed
   fresh spinach

4 cups mixed melon
   balls (cantaloupe,
   honeydew and/or
   watermelon)

1 cup zucchini ribbons*

½ cup sliced red
   bell pepper

¼ cup thinly sliced
   red onion

¼ cup red wine vinegar

2 tablespoons honey

1 tablespoon extra
   virgin olive oil

2 teaspoons lime juice

1 teaspoon
   poppy seeds

1 teaspoon dried mint

*To make ribbons, thinly slice
zucchini lengthwise with
vegetable peeler or spiral cutter.

**1.** Combine spinach, melon, zucchini, bell pepper and onion in large bowl.

**2.** Combine vinegar, honey, oil, lime juice, poppy seeds and mint in small jar with tight-fitting lid; shake well.

**3.** Pour dressing over salad; toss gently to coat.

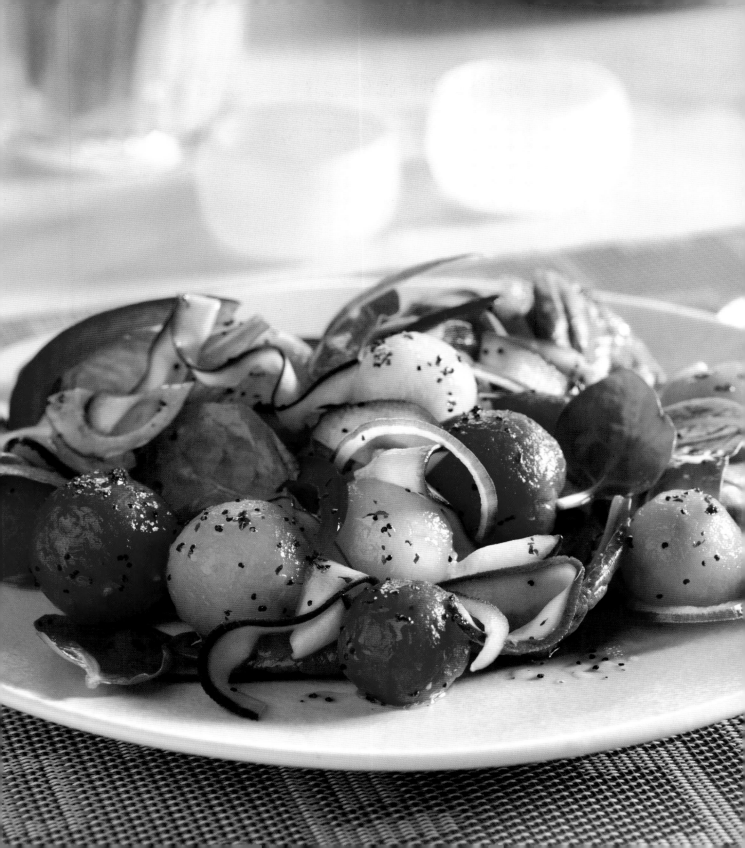

# FENNEL BRAISED WITH TOMATO

Makes 6 servings

2 bulbs fennel

1 tablespoon olive oil

1 small onion, sliced

1 clove garlic, sliced

4 medium tomatoes, chopped

⅔ cup vegetable broth or water

3 tablespoons dry white wine or vegetable broth

1 tablespoon chopped fresh marjoram *or* 1 teaspoon dried marjoram

½ teaspoon salt

¼ teaspoon black pepper

**1.** Trim stems and bottoms from fennel bulbs; reserve fronds for garnish. Cut each bulb lengthwise into four wedges.

**2.** Heat oil in large skillet over medium heat. Add fennel, onion and garlic; cook about 5 minutes or until onion is soft and translucent, stirring occasionally.

**3.** Stir in tomatoes, broth, wine, marjoram, salt and pepper; cover and cook over low heat about 20 minutes or until fennel is tender. Garnish with reserved fennel fronds.

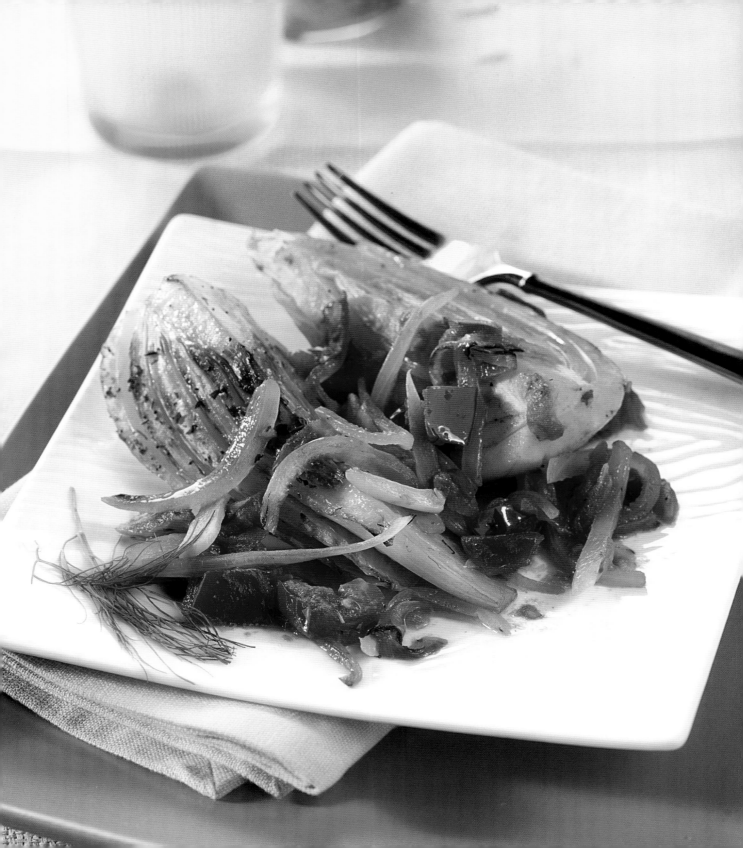

# SAUTÉED SWISS CHARD

Makes 4 servings

1 large bunch Swiss
  chard or kale
  (about 1 pound)

1 tablespoon olive oil

3 cloves garlic, minced

¾ teaspoon salt

¼ teaspoon black
  pepper

1 tablespoon balsamic
  vinegar (optional)

¼ cup pine nuts,
  toasted*

*To toast pine nuts, cook in
small skillet over medium heat
1 to 2 minutes or until lightly
browned, stirring frequently.

**1.** Rinse chard in cold water; shake off excess water but do not dry. Finely chop stems; coarsely chop leaves.

**2.** Heat oil in large saucepan over medium heat. Add garlic; cook and stir 2 minutes. Add chard, salt and pepper; cover and cook 2 minutes or until chard begins to wilt. Uncover; cook and stir 5 minutes or until chard is evenly wilted.

**3.** Stir in vinegar, if desired. Sprinkle with pine nuts just before serving.

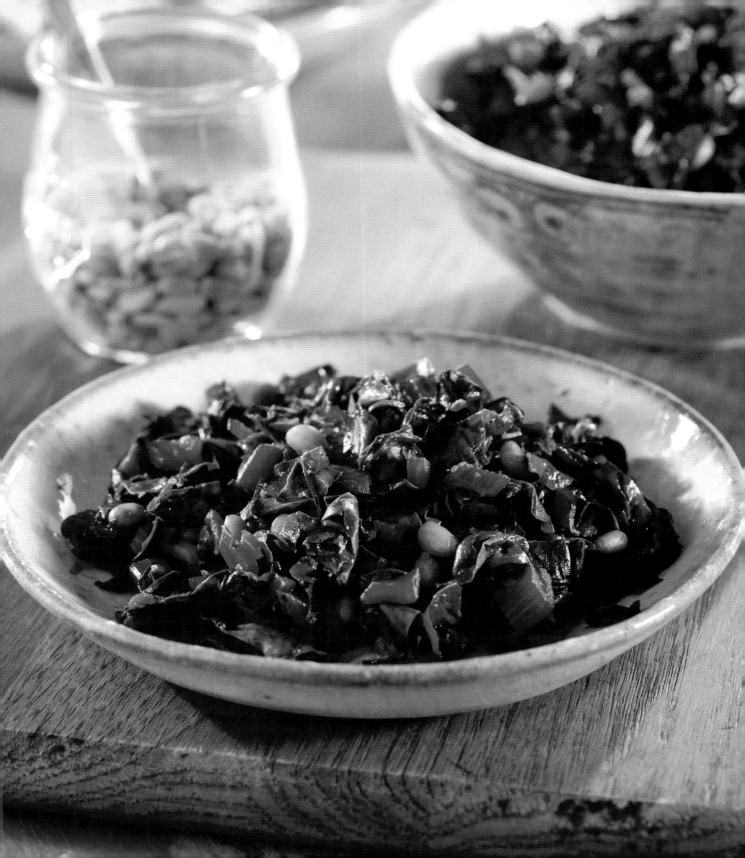

# GRILLED SESAME ASPARAGUS
Makes 4 servings

1 pound medium asparagus spears (about 20), trimmed

2 teaspoons olive oil

1 teaspoon dark sesame oil

1 tablespoon sesame seeds

2 to 3 teaspoons balsamic vinegar

¼ teaspoon salt

¼ teaspoon black pepper

**1.** Oil grid. Prepare grill for direct cooking.

**2.** Place asparagus on baking sheet; drizzle with olive oil and sesame oil. Sprinkle with sesame seeds, rolling to coat.

**3.** Grill asparagus over medium-high heat 4 to 6 minutes or until beginning to brown, turning once. Transfer to serving dish; sprinkle with vinegar, salt and pepper.

# BEET CHIPS
Makes 2 to 3 servings

3 medium beets (red and/or golden), trimmed

1½ tablespoons olive oil

¼ teaspoon salt

¼ teaspoon black pepper

**1.** Preheat oven to 300°F.

**2.** Cut beets into very thin slices (about 1/16 inch thick). Combine beets, oil, salt and pepper in medium bowl; toss gently to coat. Arrange in single layer on baking sheets.

**3.** Bake 30 to 35 minutes or until beets are darkened and crisp.* Spread on paper towels to cool completely.

*If the beet chips are darkened but not crisp, turn oven off and let chips stand in oven until crisp, about 10 minutes. Do not keep the oven on as the chips will burn easily.*

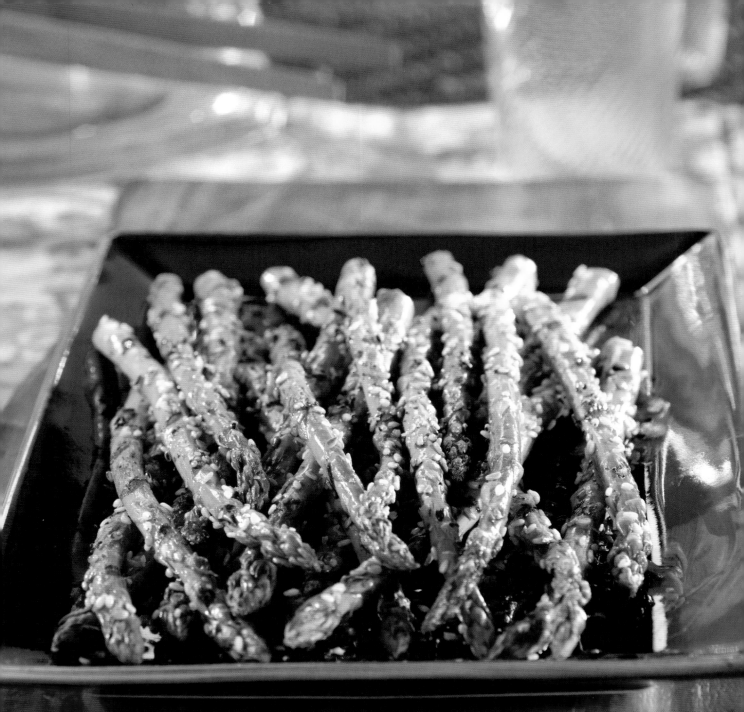

Grilled Sesame Asparagus

# CURRIED GINGER PUMPKIN SOUP

## Makes 8 servings

1 tablespoon
  coconut oil

1 large sweet onion
  (such as Walla
  Walla), coarsely
  chopped

1 large Golden
  Delicious apple,
  peeled and coarsely
  chopped

3 slices (¼ inch)
  peeled fresh ginger

1½ teaspoons
  curry powder

2½ cups chicken or
  vegetable broth,
  divided

2 cans (15 ounces each)
  solid-pack pumpkin

¾ cup canned coconut
  milk, well shaken

1 teaspoon salt

¼ teaspoon
  black pepper

Roasted salted
  pumpkin seeds
  (pepitas)

**1.** Heat oil in large saucepan over medium heat. Add onion, apple, ginger and curry powder; cook and stir 10 minutes. Add ¾ cup broth; cover and cook 10 minutes or until apple is tender.

**2.** Pour onion mixture into blender; blend until smooth. Return to saucepan. (Or use hand-held immersion blender.)

**3.** Add pumpkin, remaining 1¾ cups broth, coconut milk, salt and pepper; cook 5 minutes or until heated through, stirring occasionally. Sprinkle with pumpkin seeds, if desired.

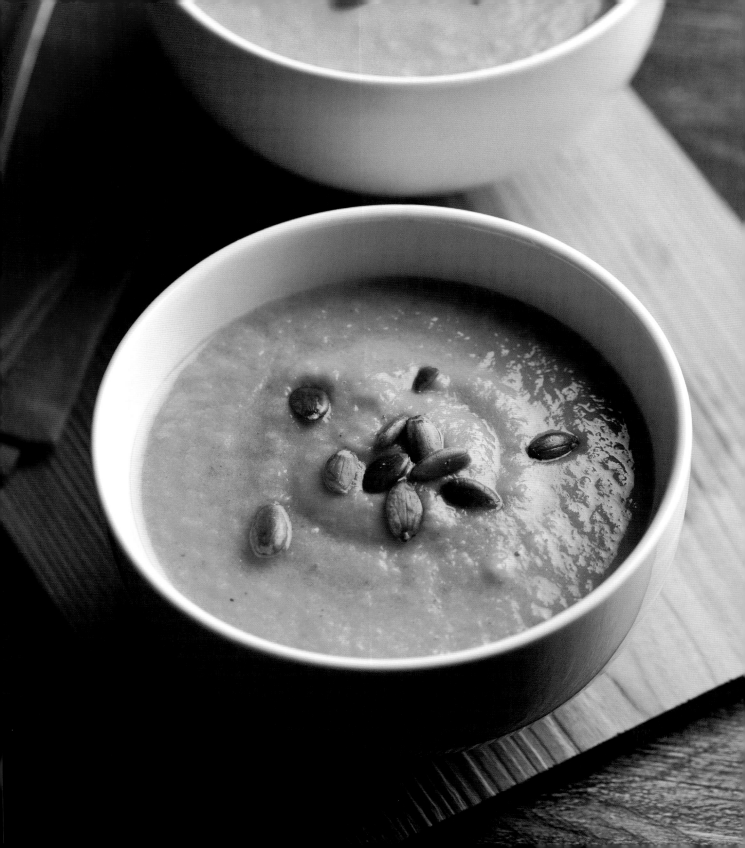

# CAULIFLOWER TABBOULEH

Makes 6 servings

2 packages (12 ounces each) cauliflower florets

3 tablespoons olive oil, divided

1 teaspoon curry powder

1 small bunch Italian parsley

1 small onion, finely chopped

½ seedless cucumber, chopped

1 cup chopped ripe tomato *or* 1 can (about 14 ounces) diced tomatoes, well drained

⅓ cup lemon juice

½ teaspoon salt

½ teaspoon black pepper

**1.** Cut large cauliflower florets into smaller. pieces. Place cauliflower in food processor; pulse 1 minute or until chopped into uniform rice-size pieces.

**2.** Heat 1 tablespoon oil in large skillet over medium-high heat. Add curry powder; cook until sizzling. Add cauliflower; cook 10 minutes, stirring frequently. Set aside to cool.

**3.** Meanwhile, trim and discard large stems from parsley. Place parsley sprigs in food processor; pulse 10 to 20 seconds until chopped.

**4.** Combine cauliflower, parsley, onion, cucumber and tomato in large bowl. Whisk remaining 2 tablespoons oil, lemon juice, salt and pepper in small bowl until well blended.

**5.** Pour dressing over cauliflower mixture; toss to coat. Serve at room temperature or chilled.

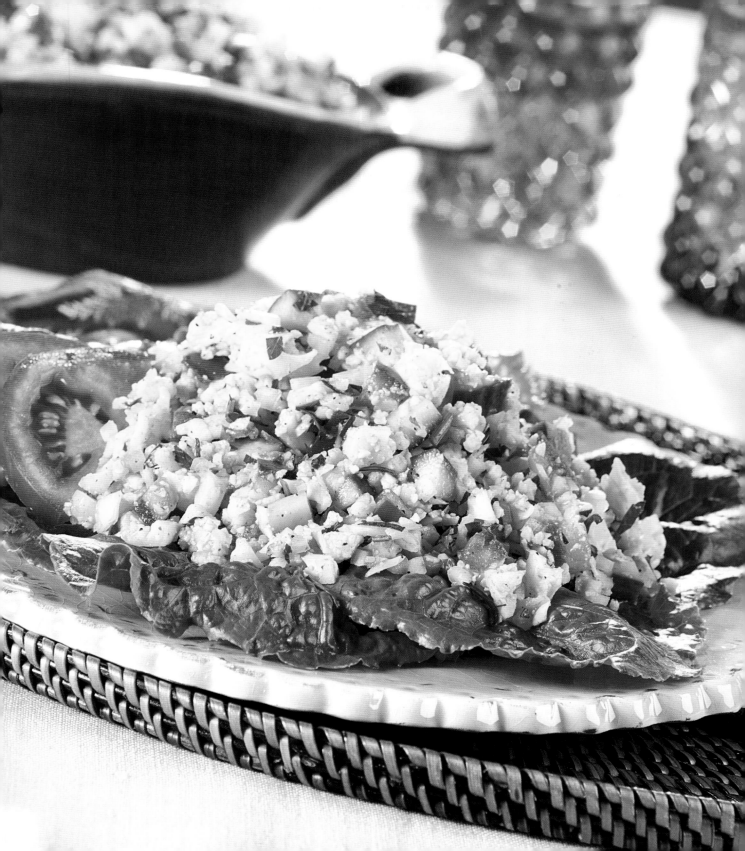

# MARINATED TOMATO SALAD

Makes 6 to 8 servings

2 cups cherry
   tomatoes,
   cut into halves

1 large cucumber, cut
   in half lengthwise
   and sliced

1 large yellow or
   red bell pepper,
   cut into strips

3 slices red onion,
   quartered

2 tablespoons
   balsamic vinegar

1 tablespoon olive oil

½ teaspoon salt

½ teaspoon dried basil

¼ teaspoon
   garlic powder

¼ teaspoon
   dried oregano

**1.** Combine tomatoes, cucumber, bell pepper and onion in large bowl.

**2.** Combine vinegar, oil, salt, basil, garlic powder and oregano in small bowl; mix well.

**3.** Pour dressing over vegetables; toss to coat. Serve immediately or cover and refrigerate 2 hours for flavors to blend.

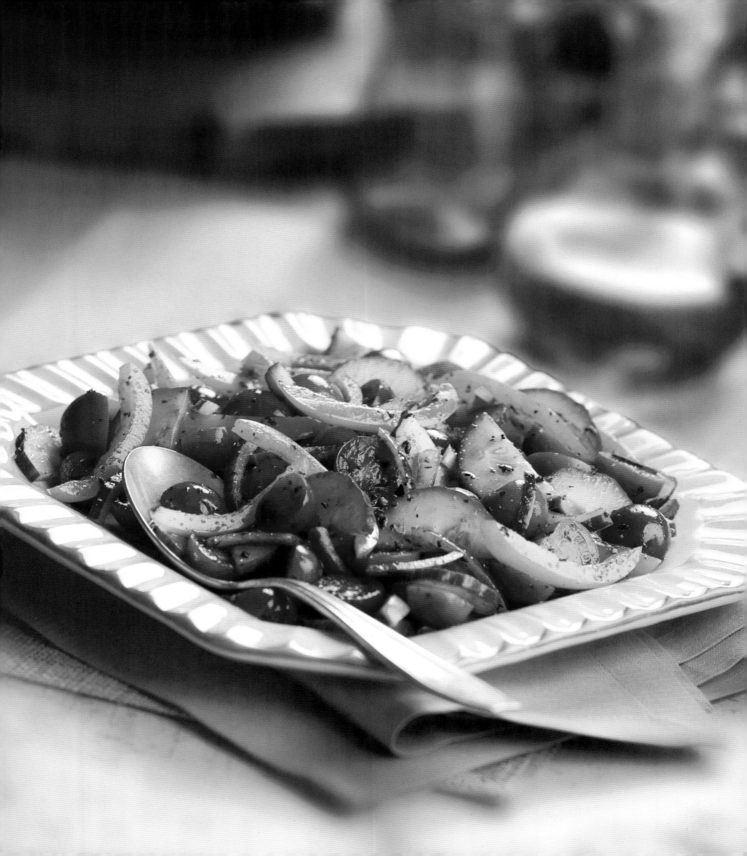

# SAVORY PUMPKIN HUMMUS

Makes 1½ cups

1 can (15 ounces) solid-pack pumpkin

3 tablespoons chopped fresh parsley, plus additional for garnish

3 tablespoons tahini

3 tablespoons lemon juice

3 cloves garlic

1 teaspoon ground cumin

½ teaspoon salt

⅛ teaspoon black pepper

⅛ teaspoon ground red pepper, plus additional for garnish

Assorted vegetable sticks

1. Combine pumpkin, 3 tablespoons parsley, tahini, lemon juice, garlic, cumin, salt, black pepper and ⅛ teaspoon red pepper in food processor or blender; process until smooth. Cover and refrigerate at least 2 hours to allow flavors to blend.

2. Sprinkle with additional red pepper, if desired. Garnish with additional parsley. Serve with assorted vegetable sticks.

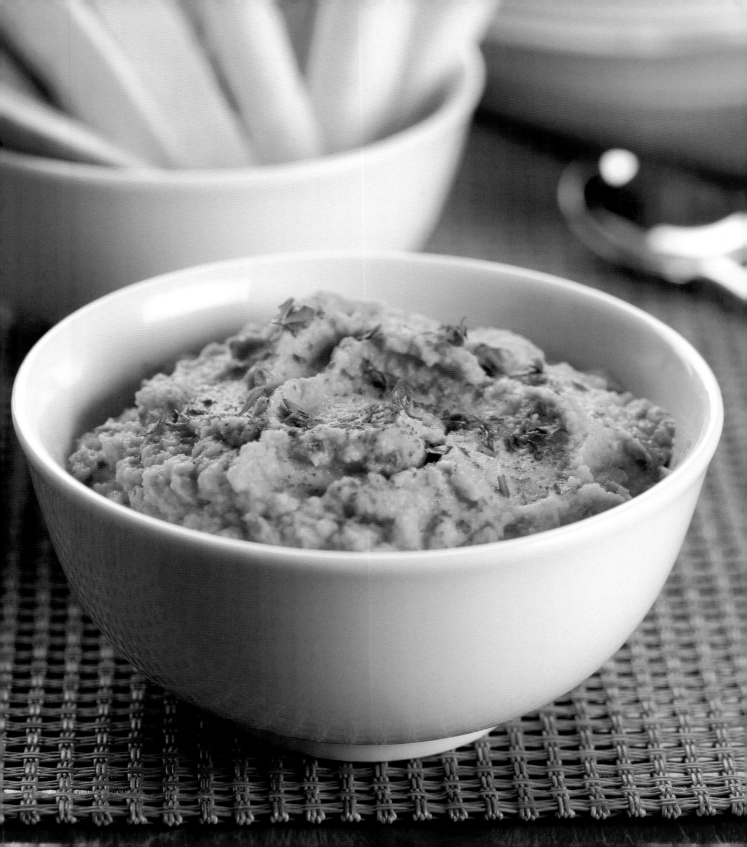

# SKILLET ROASTED ROOT VEGETABLES

Makes 4 servings

 1 sweet potato,
    peeled, cut in half
    lengthwise and
    cut crosswise
    into ½-inch slices

 1 large red onion, cut
    into 1-inch wedges

 2 parsnips, cut
    diagonally into
    1-inch slices

 2 carrots, cut
    diagonally into
    1-inch slices

 1 turnip, peeled, cut
    in half and then cut
    into ½-inch slices

2½ tablespoons olive oil

1½ tablespoons honey

1½ tablespoons
    balsamic vinegar

 1 teaspoon coarse salt

 1 teaspoon
    dried thyme

 ¼ teaspoon ground
    red pepper

 ¼ teaspoon
    black pepper

**1.** Preheat oven to 400°F.

**2.** Combine all ingredients in large bowl; toss to coat. Spread vegetables in single layer in large cast iron skillet.

**3.** Roast 1 hour or until vegetables are tender, stirring once halfway through cooking time.

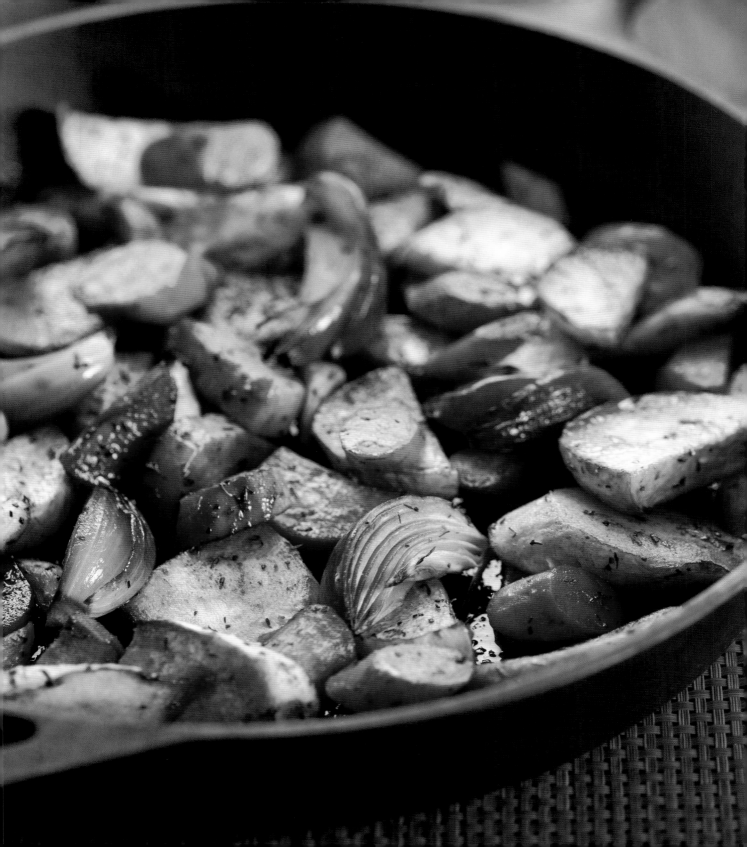

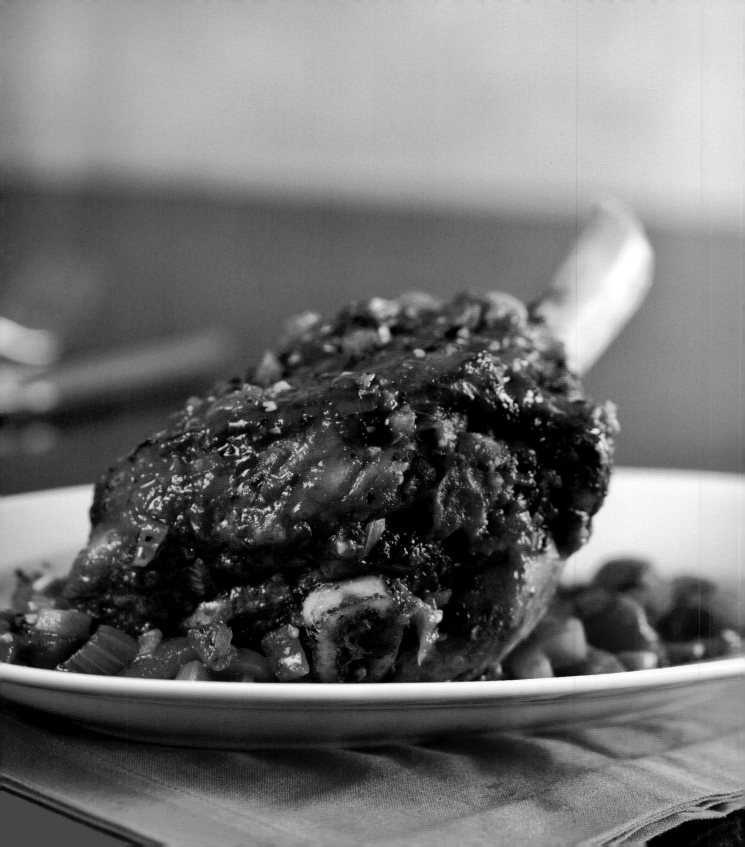

# PALEO SLOW

## BRAISED LAMB SHANKS
### Makes 4 servings

4 lamb shanks (12 to 16 ounces each)

¾ teaspoon salt, divided

¼ teaspoon black pepper

1 tablespoon olive oil

1 medium onion, chopped

2 stalks celery, chopped

2 carrots, chopped

6 cloves garlic, minced

1 teaspoon dried basil

1 can (about 14 ounces) diced tomatoes

2 tablespoons tomato paste

Chopped fresh Italian parsley (optional)

**1.** Season lamb with ½ teaspoon salt and pepper. Heat oil in large skillet over medium-high heat. Add lamb; cook 8 to 10 minutes or until browned on all sides. Transfer to slow cooker.

**2.** Add onion, celery, carrots, garlic and basil to skillet; cook and stir 4 minutes or until vegetables are softened. Add tomatoes, tomato paste and remaining ¼ teaspoon salt; cook and stir 2 to 3 minutes or until slightly thickened. Pour mixture over lamb in slow cooker.

**3.** Cover; cook on LOW 8 to 9 hours or until lamb is very tender. Remove lamb to large serving platter; tent with foil.

**4.** Turn slow cooker to HIGH. Cook, uncovered, 10 to 15 minutes or until sauce is thickened. Serve lamb with sauce; garnish with parsley.

# MAPLE SPICE RUBBED RIBS

## Makes 4 servings

2 teaspoons chili powder, divided

1 teaspoon ground coriander

1 teaspoon garlic powder, divided

½ teaspoon salt

¼ teaspoon black pepper

3 to 3½ pounds pork baby back ribs, trimmed and cut in half

3 tablespoons maple syrup, divided

1 can (8 ounces) tomato sauce

¼ teaspoon ground cinnamon

¼ teaspoon ground ginger

**1.** Combine 1 teaspoon chili powder, coriander, ½ teaspoon garlic powder, salt and pepper in small bowl; mix well. Brush ribs with 1 tablespoon maple syrup; sprinkle with spice mixture. Transfer to slow cooker.

**2.** Combine tomato sauce, remaining 1 teaspoon chili powder, ½ teaspoon garlic powder, 2 tablespoons maple syrup, cinnamon and ginger in medium bowl; mix well. Pour over ribs in slow cooker.

**3.** Cover; cook on LOW 8 to 9 hours. Remove ribs to large platter; tent with foil.

**4.** Turn slow cooker to HIGH. Cover; cook 10 to 15 minutes or until sauce is thickened. Brush ribs with sauce; serve any remaining sauce on the side.

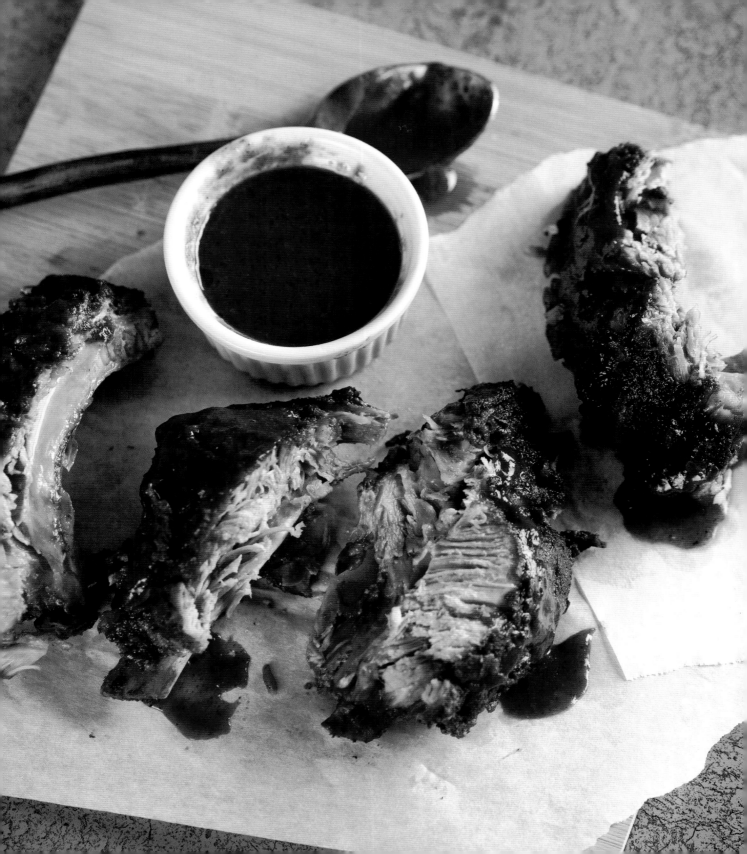

# CREAMY SWEET POTATO AND BUTTERNUT SQUASH SOUP

Makes 4 to 6 servings

1 pound sweet
   potatoes, cut
   into 1-inch pieces

1 pound butternut
   squash, cut into
   1-inch pieces

1 can (about 14 ounces)
   chicken broth,
   divided

½ cup chopped onion

1 can (about 13 ounces)
   coconut milk

1½ teaspoons salt

½ teaspoon
   ground cumin

½ teaspoon ground
   red pepper

1 to 2 green onions,
   finely chopped
   (optional)

**1.** Combine sweet potatoes, squash, half of broth and onion in slow cooker.

**2.** Cover; cook on HIGH 4 hours or until vegetables are tender.

**3.** Process sweet potato mixture, 1 cup at a time, in food processor or blender until smooth. (Or use hand-held immersion blender.) Return to slow cooker; stir in remaining broth, coconut milk, salt, cumin and red pepper.

**4.** Cover; cook on HIGH 15 minutes or until heated through. Sprinkle with green onions, if desired.

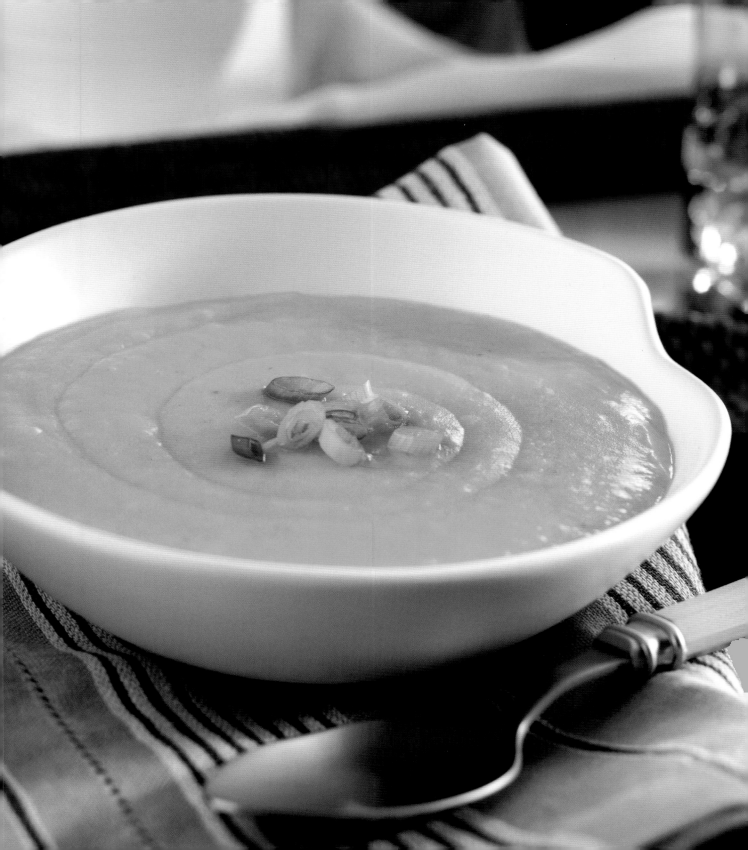

# PORK ROAST WITH CURRANT CHERRY SALSA

Makes 6 to 8 servings

1½ teaspoons
   chili powder

¾ teaspoon salt

½ teaspoon
   garlic powder

½ teaspoon paprika

¼ teaspoon
   ground allspice

1 boneless pork loin
   roast (2 pounds)

1 tablespoon olive oil

½ cup water

1 package (1 pound)
   frozen pitted dark
   cherries, thawed,
   drained and halved

¼ cup currants or
   dark raisins

1 teaspoon grated
   orange peel

1 teaspoon
   balsamic vinegar

⅛ to ¼ teaspoon red
   pepper flakes

**1.** Combine chili powder, salt, garlic powder, paprika and allspice in small bowl; mix well. Rub mixture over all sides of pork.

**2.** Heat oil in large skillet over medium-high heat. Add pork; cook 6 to 8 minutes or until browned on all sides. Transfer to slow cooker.

**3.** Stir water into skillet, scraping up browned bits from bottom of skillet. Pour into slow cooker around pork.

**4.** Cover; cook on LOW 6 to 8 hours. Remove pork to cutting board; tent with foil. Let stand 10 to 15 minutes. Strain juices from slow cooker into bowl; discard solids. Keep warm.

**5.** Turn slow cooker to HIGH. Add cherries, currants, orange peel, vinegar and red pepper flakes to slow cooker. Cover; cook 30 minutes. Slice pork; spoon warm juices over meat. Serve with salsa.

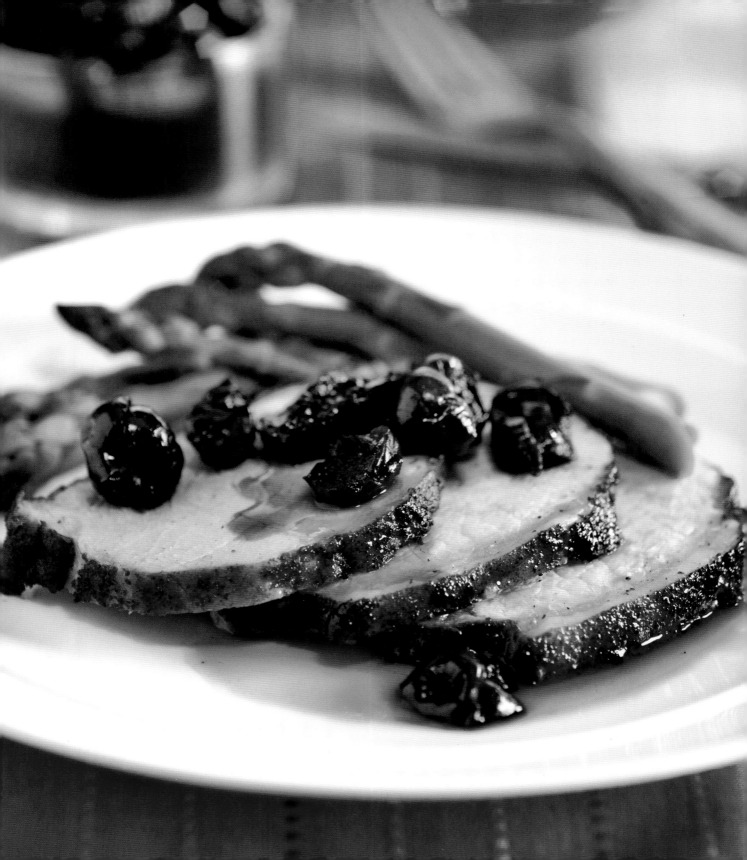

# BEEF AND BEET BORSCHT

Makes 6 to 8 servings

6 slices bacon

1 boneless beef chuck roast (1½ pounds), trimmed and cut into ½-inch pieces

1 medium onion, chopped

4 cloves garlic, minced

3 cups beef broth

4 medium beets, peeled and cut into ½-inch pieces

2 large carrots, sliced

6 sprigs fresh dill

3 tablespoons honey

3 tablespoons red wine vinegar

2 bay leaves

3 cups shredded green cabbage

**1.** Cook bacon in large skillet over medium heat until crisp. Remove to paper towel-lined plate. Crumble bacon.

**2.** Add beef to skillet; cook 5 minutes or until browned, stirring occationally. Transfer to slow cooker.

**3.** Pour off all but 1 tablespoon fat from skillet. Add onion and garlic; cook and stir 3 minutes or until onion is softened. Transfer to slow cooker. Stir in broth, beets, carrots, bacon, dill, honey, vinegar and bay leaves; mix well.

**4.** Cover; cook on LOW 5 to 6 hours. Stir in cabbage. Cover; cook on LOW 30 minutes. Remove and discard bay leaves before serving.

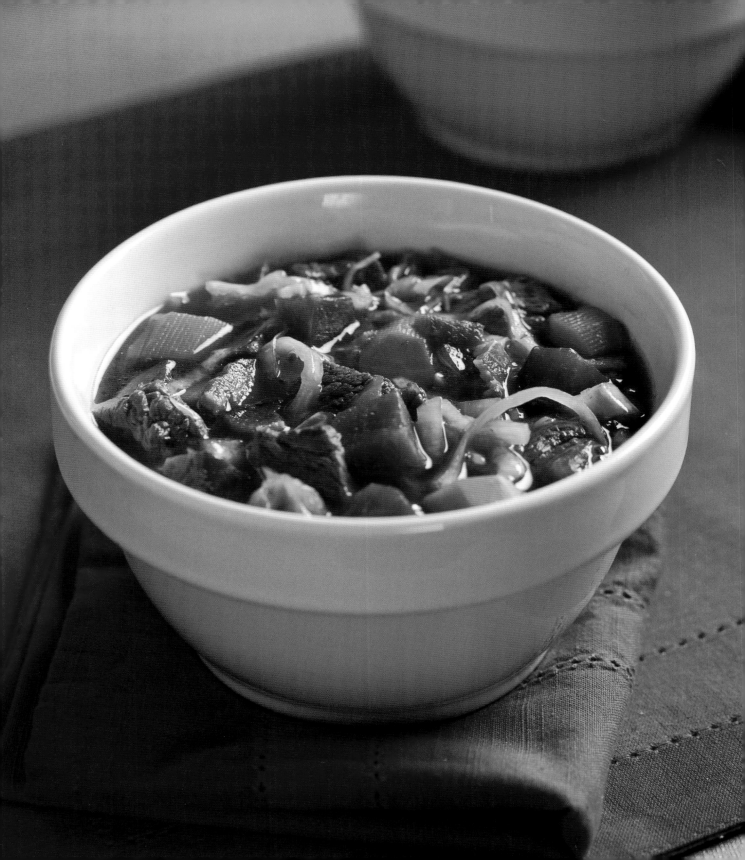

# PULLED PORK WITH HONEY-CHIPOTLE BARBECUE SAUCE

Makes 8 servings

1 tablespoon chili powder, divided

1 teaspoon chipotle chili powder, divided

1 teaspoon ground cumin, divided

1 teaspoon garlic powder, divided

1 teaspoon salt

1 bone-in pork shoulder (3½ pounds), trimmed

1 can (15 ounces) tomato sauce

5 tablespoons honey, divided

**1.** Combine 1 teaspoon chili powder, ½ teaspoon chipotle chili powder, ½ teaspoon cumin, ½ teaspoon garlic powder and salt in small bowl; mix well. Rub spice mixture over all sides of pork. Place pork in slow cooker.

**2.** Combine tomato sauce, 4 tablespoons honey, remaining 2 teaspoons chili powder, ½ teaspoon chipotle chili powder, ½ teaspoon cumin and ½ teaspoon garlic powder in large bowl; mix well. Pour over pork in slow cooker.

**3.** Cover; cook on LOW 8 hours. Remove pork to large bowl; tent with foil.

**4.** Turn slow cooker to HIGH. Cover; cook 30 minutes or until sauce is thickened. Stir in remaining 1 tablespoon honey. Turn off heat.

**5.** Remove bone from pork; shred meat into bite-size pieces with two forks. Stir shredded pork back into slow cooker to coat with sauce.

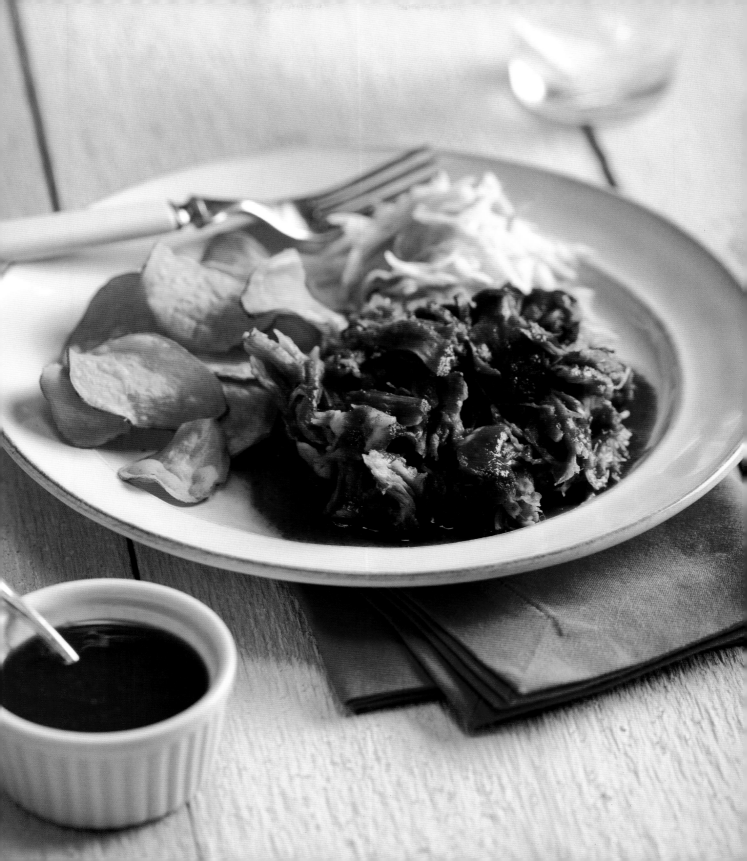

# INDIAN-STYLE APRICOT CHICKEN

Makes 4 to 6 servings

6 skinless chicken thighs (about 2 pounds)

½ teaspoon salt

¼ teaspoon black pepper

1 tablespoon coconut oil

1 large onion, chopped

2 tablespoons grated fresh ginger

2 cloves garlic, minced

½ teaspoon ground cinnamon

⅛ teaspoon ground allspice

1 can (about 14 ounces) diced tomatoes

1 cup chicken broth

1 package (8 ounces) dried apricots

Pinch saffron threads (optional)

Hot cooked basmati rice

Chopped fresh Italian parsley (optional)

**1.** Season chicken with ½ teaspoon salt and ¼ teaspoon pepper. Heat oil in large skillet over medium-high heat. Add chicken; cook until browned on all sides. Transfer to slow cooker.

**2.** Add onion to skillet; cook and stir 3 to 5 minutes or until translucent. Stir in ginger, garlic, cinnamon and allspice; cook and stir 30 seconds or until fragrant. Stir in tomatoes and broth; cook 2 minutes, scraping up browned bits from bottom of skillet. Pour into slow cooker. Add apricots and saffron, if desired.

**3.** Cover; cook on LOW 5 to 6 hours or on HIGH 3 to 4 hours. Season with additional salt and pepper, if desired. Serve with basmati rice; garnish with parsley.

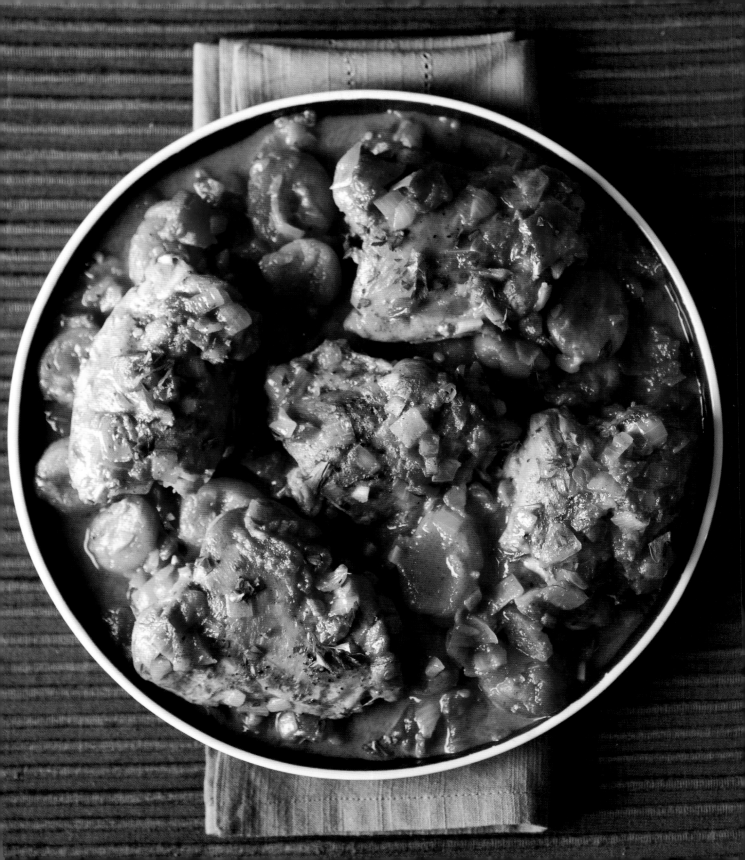

# POT ROAST WITH BACON AND MUSHROOMS

### Makes 6 to 8 servings

6 slices bacon

1 boneless beef chuck roast (2½ to 3 pounds), trimmed*

¾ teaspoon salt, divided

¼ teaspoon black pepper

¾ cup chopped shallots

8 ounces sliced mushrooms

¼ ounce dried porcini mushrooms (optional)

4 cloves garlic, minced

1 teaspoon dried oregano

1 cup beef broth

2 tablespoons tomato paste

Roasted Cauliflower (recipe follows, optional)

*Unless you have a 5-, 6- or 7-quart slow cooker, cut any roast larger than 2½ pounds in half so it cooks completely.*

**1.** Cook bacon in large skillet over medium heat until crisp. Remove to paper towel-lined plate. Crumble bacon.

**2.** Pour off all but 2 tablespoons drippings from skillet. Season beef with ½ teaspoon salt and pepper. Add beef to skillet; cook 8 minutes or until well browned on all sides. Remove to large plate. Add shallots, sliced mushrooms, porcini mushrooms, if desired, garlic, oregano and remaining ¼ teaspoon salt to skillet; cook and stir 3 to 4 minutes or until vegetables are softened. Stir in bacon. Transfer to slow cooker.

**3.** Place beef on top of vegetables in slow cooker. Combine broth and tomato paste in small bowl; mix well. Pour over beef.

**4.** Cover; cook on LOW 8 hours. Prepare Roasted Cauliflower, if desired.

**5.** Remove beef to cutting board; tent with foil. Let stand 10 minutes before slicing. Serve beef with vegetables, cooking liquid and Roasted Cauliflower, if desired.

**ROASTED CAULIFLOWER:** Preheat oven to 375°F. Break 1 head cauliflower into florets onto large baking sheet. Drizzle with 2 tablespoons olive oil; sprinkle with ½ teaspoon salt and toss to coat. Roast 20 minutes; turn and roast 20 minutes or until tender and lightly browned.

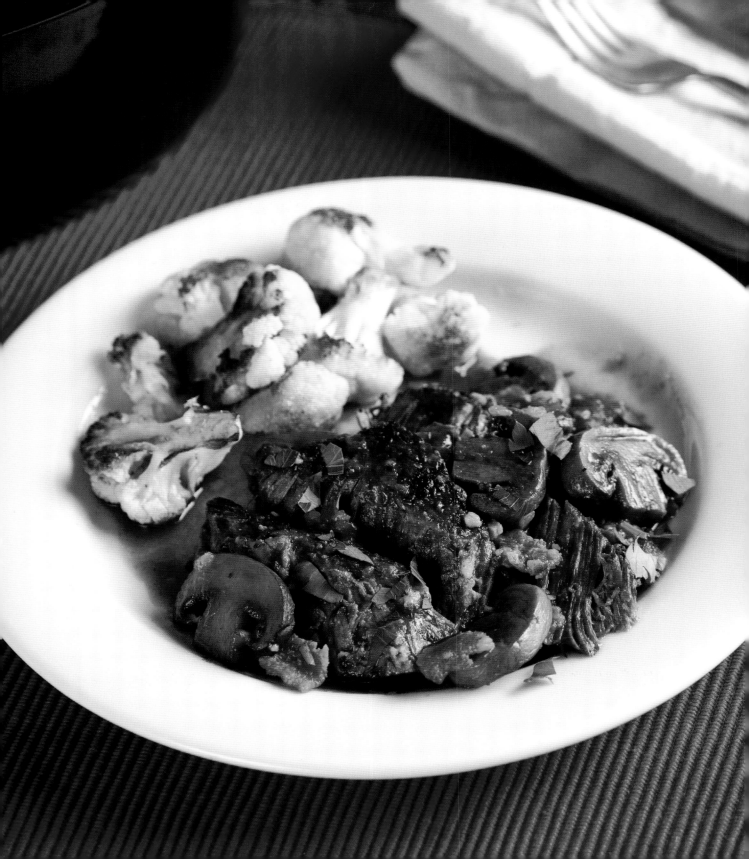

# MEDITERRANEAN MEATBALL RATATOUILLE

Makes 6 servings

1 pound bulk mild
   Italian sausage

1 package (8 ounces)
   sliced mushrooms

1 small eggplant, diced

1 zucchini, diced

½ cup chopped onion

1 clove garlic, minced

1 teaspoon dried
   oregano, divided

1 teaspoon salt,
   divided

½ teaspoon black
   pepper, divided

2 tomatoes, diced

1 tablespoon
   tomato paste

2 tablespoons
   chopped fresh basil

1 teaspoon lemon juice

**1.** Shape sausage into 1-inch meatballs. Brown meatballs in large skillet over medium heat.

**2.** Place half of meatballs in slow cooker; top with half each of mushrooms, eggplant and zucchini. Top with onion, garlic, ½ teaspoon oregano, ½ teaspoon salt and ¼ teaspoon pepper.

**3.** Add remaining meatballs, mushrooms, eggplant, zucchini, ½ teaspoon oregano, ½ teaspoon salt and ¼ teaspoon pepper.

**4.** Cover; cook on LOW 6 to 7 hours. Stir in tomatoes and tomato paste Cover; cook on LOW 15 minutes. Stir in basil and lemon juice just before serving.

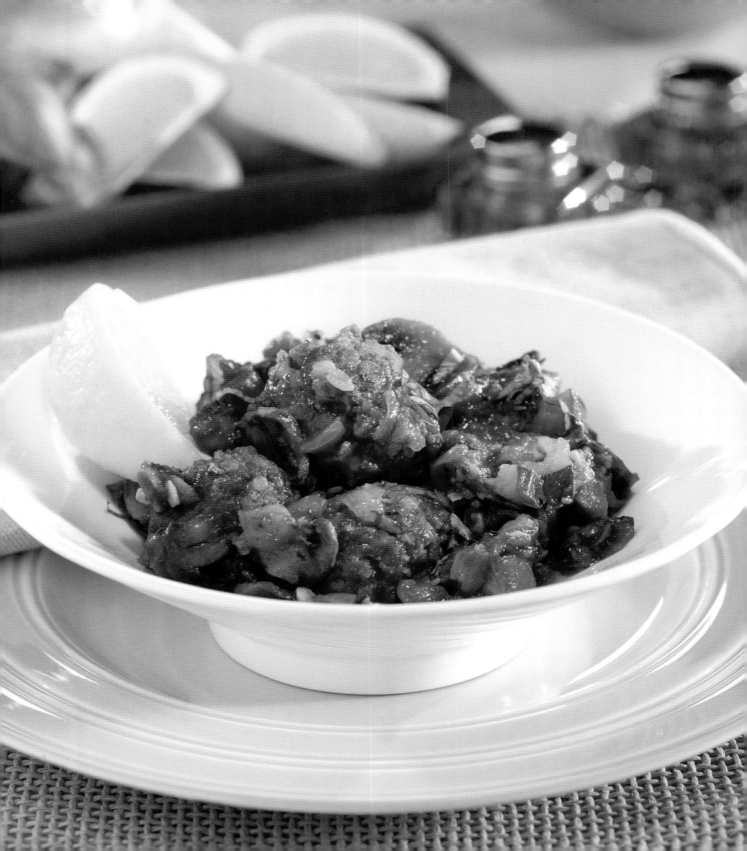

# BRAISED SHORT RIBS WITH AROMATIC SPICES

Makes 4 servings

3 pounds bone-in beef short ribs, trimmed

1 teaspoon ground cumin, divided

1 teaspoon salt

½ teaspoon black pepper

1 tablespoon olive oil

2 medium onions, halved and thinly sliced

10 cloves garlic, thinly sliced

2 tablespoons balsamic vinegar

2 tablespoons honey

1 whole cinnamon stick

2 whole star anise pods

2 large sweet potatoes, peeled and cut into ¾-inch pieces

1 cup beef broth

**1.** Season short ribs with ½ teaspoon cumin, salt and pepper. Heat oil in large skillet over medium-high heat. Add short ribs; cook 8 minutes or until browned, turning occasionally. Remove to large plate.

**2.** Add onions and garlic to skillet; cook 12 to 14 minutes or until onions are lightly browned, stirring occasionally. Add vinegar; cook and stir 1 minute. Add remaining ½ teaspoon cumin, honey, cinnamon stick and star anise; cook and stir 30 seconds. Transfer to slow cooker. Stir in sweet potatoes; top with short ribs. Pour in broth.

**3.** Cover; cook on LOW 8 to 9 hours or until meat is falling off the bones.

**4.** Remove and discard bones, cinnamon stick and star anise. Turn off heat; let stand 5 to 10 minutes. Skim off and discard fat. Serve short ribs with sauce and vegetables.

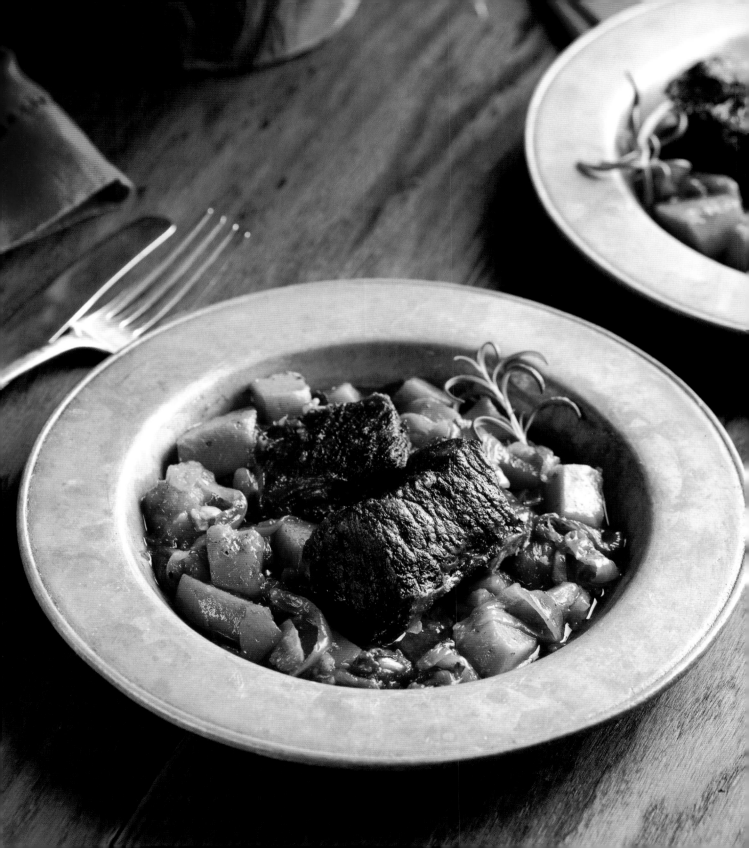

# MIDDLE EASTERN BEEF AND EGGPLANT STEW

Makes 4 servings

1 tablespoon olive oil

1 small eggplant, cut into 1-inch pieces

2 cups shiitake or cremini mushrooms, quartered

1 can (about 14 ounces) diced tomatoes

8 ounces boneless beef top round steak, cut into 1-inch pieces

1 medium onion, chopped

1 cup beef broth

Grated peel of 1 lemon

1 clove garlic, minced

½ teaspoon salt

⅓ teaspoon ground cumin

¼ teaspoon red pepper flakes

¼ teaspoon ground cinnamon

⅛ teaspoon black pepper

**1.** Heat oil in large skillet over medium-high heat. Add eggplant; cook 3 to 5 minutes or until lightly browned on all sides, stirring occasionally. Transfer to slow cooker.

**2.** Stir in mushrooms, tomatoes, beef, onion, broth, lemon peel, garlic, salt, cumin, red pepper flakes, cinnamon and black pepper; mix well.

**3.** Cover; cook on LOW 6 hours.

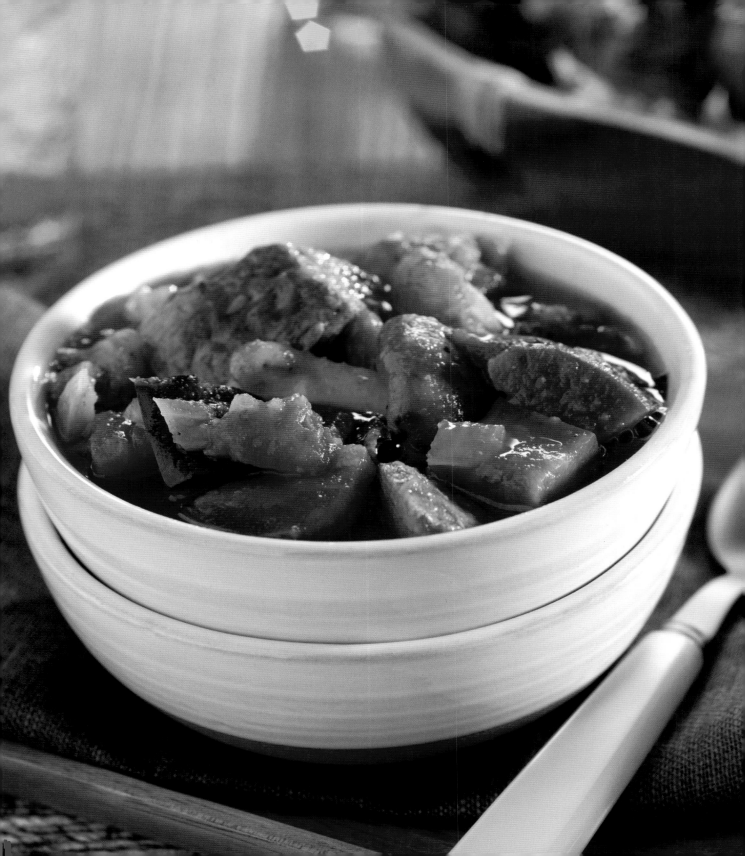

# PORK PICADILLO

Makes 4 servings

1 tablespoon olive oil

1 onion, chopped

2 cloves garlic, minced

1 pound boneless pork country-style ribs, trimmed and cut into 1-inch cubes

1 can (about 14 ounces) diced tomatoes

3 tablespoons cider vinegar

2 canned chipotle peppers in adobo sauce, chopped

½ cup raisins

½ teaspoon salt

½ teaspoon ground cumin

½ teaspoon ground cinnamon

**1.** Heat oil in large skillet over medium-low heat. Add onion and garlic; cook and stir 4 minutes. Add pork; cook and stir 5 to 7 minutes or until browned. Transfer to slow cooker.

**2.** Combine tomatoes, vinegar, chipotle peppers, raisins, salt, cumin and cinnamon in medium bowl; mix well. Pour over pork in slow cooker.

**3.** Cover; cook on LOW 5 hours or on HIGH 3 hours. Stir pork mixture with tongs, shredding meat into smaller pieces.

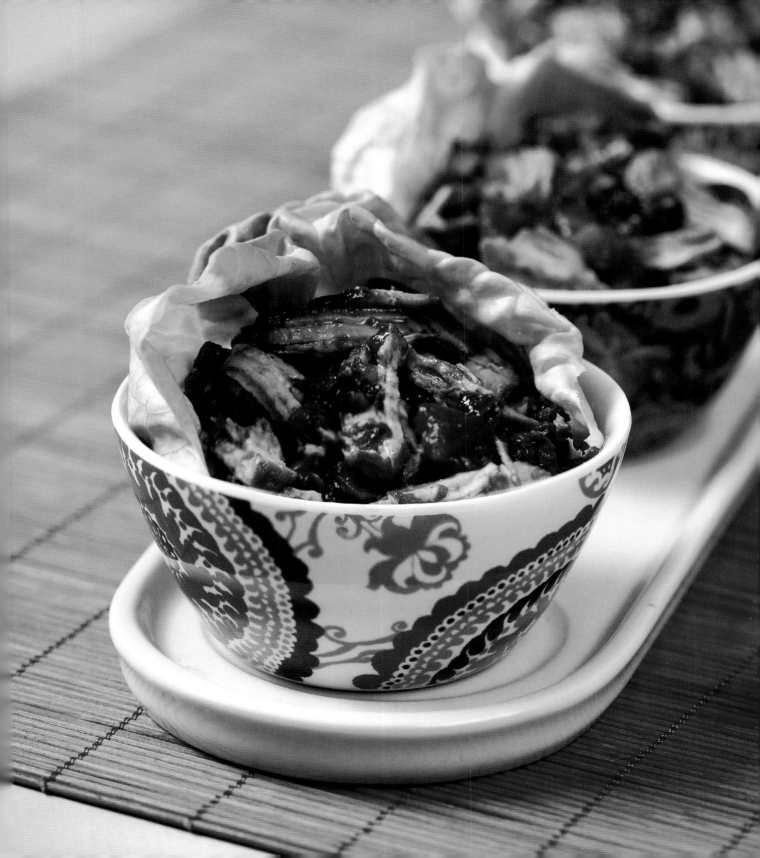

# SPICY TURKEY WITH CITRUS AU JUS

Makes 6 to 8 servings

¼ cup (½ stick)
   butter, softened

Grated peel
   of 1 lemon

1 teaspoon
   chili powder

½ teaspoon salt

¼ teaspoon
   black pepper

⅛ to ¼ teaspoon
   red pepper flakes

1 bone-in turkey breast,
   patted dry (about
   4 pounds)

1 tablespoon
   lemon juice

**1.** Combine butter, lemon peel, chili powder, ½ teaspoon salt, ¼ teaspoon black pepper and red pepper flakes in small bowl; mix well. Spread mixture over top and sides of turkey. Place turkey in slow cooker.

**2.** Cover; cook on LOW 4 to 5 hours or on HIGH 2½ to 3 hours.

**3.** Turn off heat. Remove turkey to cutting board; tent with foil. Let stand 10 to 15 minutes before slicing.

**4.** Let cooking liquid stand 5 minutes; skim off and discard fat. Stir in lemon juice; season with additional salt and black pepper. Serve turkey with sauce.

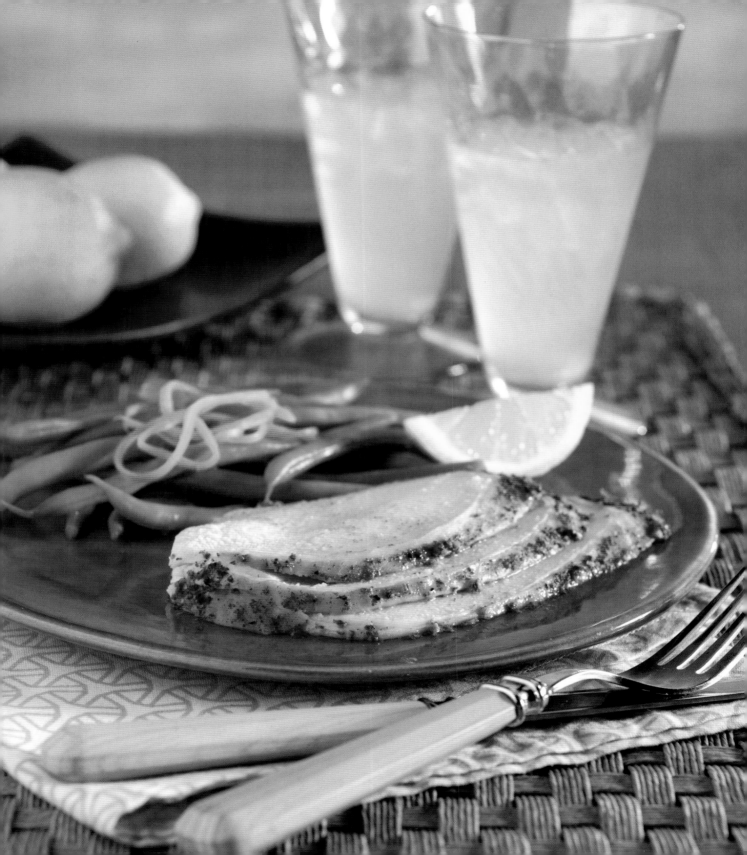

# BRAISED CHIPOTLE BEEF

Makes 4 to 6 servings

3 pounds boneless beef chuck roast, cut into 2-inch pieces

2 teaspoons salt, divided

¾ teaspoon black pepper, divided

3 tablespoons olive oil, divided

1 large onion, cut into 1-inch pieces

2 red bell peppers, cut into 1-inch pieces

3 tablespoons tomato paste

1 tablespoon minced garlic

1 tablespoon chipotle chili powder

1 tablespoon paprika

1 tablespoon ground cumin

1 teaspoon dried oregano

1 cup beef broth

1 can (about 14 ounces) diced tomatoes, drained

**1.** Pat beef dry with paper towels; season with ½ teaspoon salt and ¼ teaspoon black pepper. Heat 2 tablespoons oil in large skillet over medium-high heat. Add beef in two batches; cook until browned on all sides. Transfer to slow cooker.

**2.** Add remaining 1 tablespoon oil to skillet. Add onion; cook and stir 3 minutes or until softened. Add bell peppers; cook and stir 2 minutes. Add tomato paste, garlic, chili powder, paprika, cumin, oregano, remaining 1½ teaspoons salt and ½ teaspoon black pepper; cook and stir 1 minute. Transfer to slow cooker.

**3.** Add broth to skillet; cook 2 minutes over medium heat, scraping up browned bits from bottom of skillet. Pour over beef in slow cooker. Stir in tomatoes.

**4.** Cover; cook on LOW 7 hours. Turn off heat. Let stand 5 minutes; skim off and discard fat.

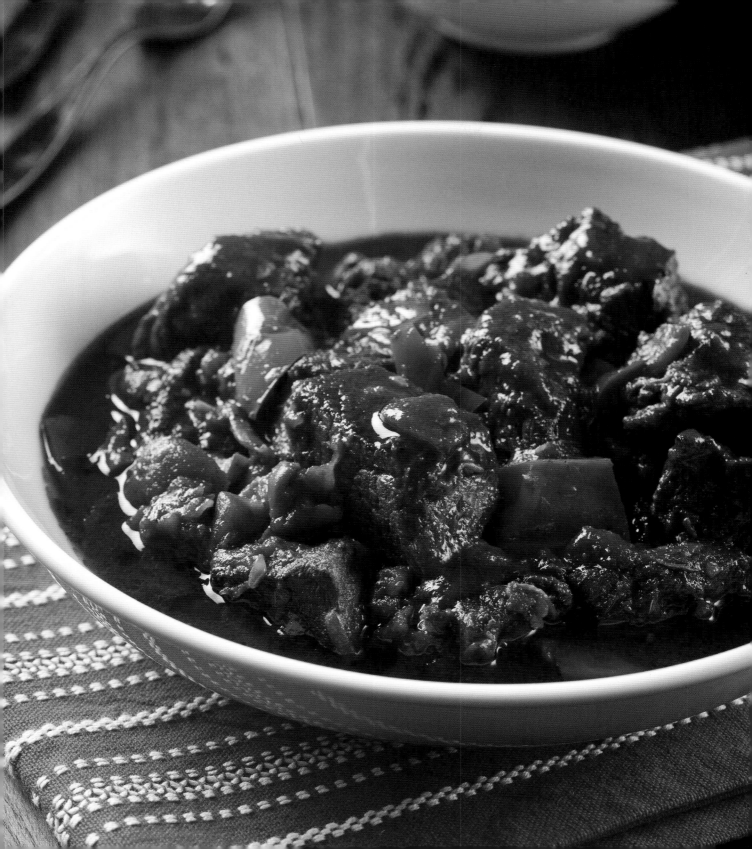

# PORK IN CHILE SAUCE

Makes 4 servings

2 large tomatoes, chopped

2 cups tomato purée

2 small poblano peppers, seeded and chopped

2 large shallots *or* 1 small onion, chopped

2 cloves garlic, minced

1 teaspoon salt

½ teaspoon dried oregano

¼ teaspoon chipotle chili powder

¼ teaspoon black pepper

2 boneless pork chops (about 6 ounces each), cut into 1-inch pieces

Almond flour tortillas or coconut wraps (optional)

**1.** Combine tomatoes, tomato purée, poblano peppers, shallots, garlic, salt, oregano, chipotle chili powder and black pepper in slow cooker; mix well. Stir in pork.

**2.** Cover; cook on LOW 5 to 6 hours. Serve with tortillas, if desired.

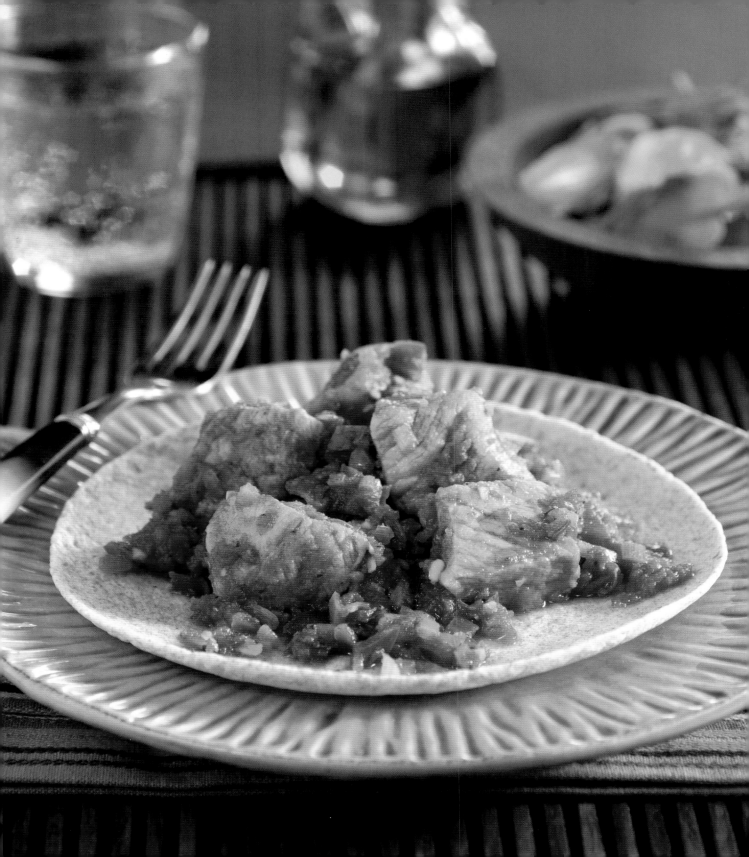

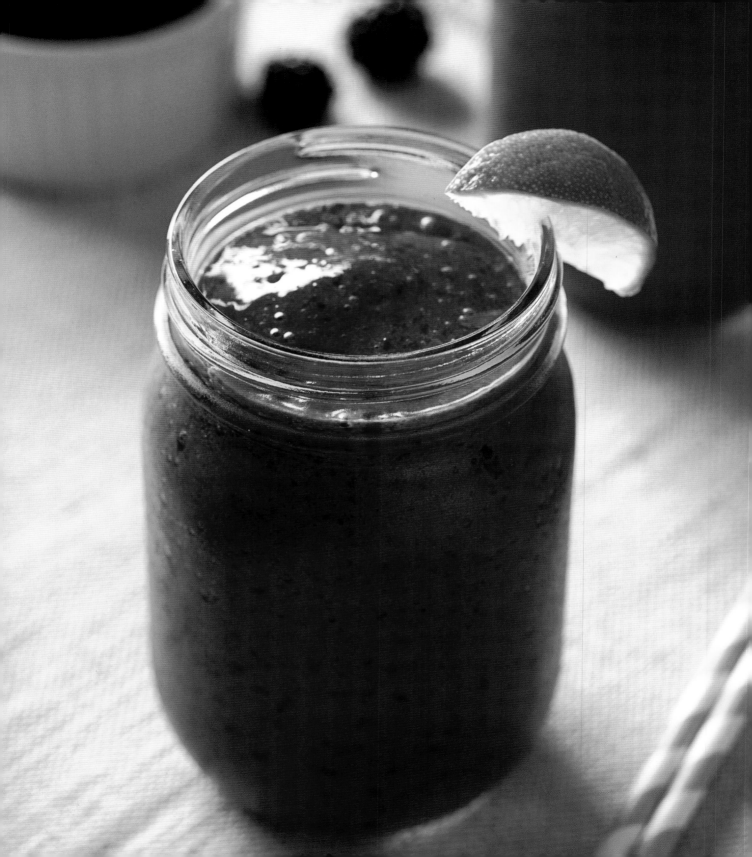

# PALEO SMOOTHIES

## BLACKBERRY LIME SMOOTHIE

Makes 1 serving

½ cup unsweetened coconut milk beverage

1 cup fresh blackberries

2 ice cubes

1 tablespoon lime juice

2 teaspoons honey

½ teaspoon grated lime peel

Combine coconut milk, blackberries, ice, lime juice, honey and lime peel in blender; blend until smooth.

# CARROT CAKE SMOOTHIE
### Makes 1 serving

½ cup coconut water

3 medium carrots, peeled and cut into chunks (about 6 ounces)

½ banana

½ cup frozen pineapple chunks

1 teaspoon honey

⅛ teaspoon ground cinnamon

⅛ teaspoon ground ginger

Combine coconut water, carrots, banana, pineapple, honey, cinnamon and ginger in blender; blend until smooth.

# GREEN ISLANDER SMOOTHIE
### Makes 2 servings

2 cups ice cubes

1½ cups fresh pineapple chunks

1 banana

1 cup packed stemmed spinach

1 cup packed stemmed kale

Combine ice, pineapple, banana, spinach and kale in blender; blend until smooth.

Carrot Cake Smoothie

# KIWI GREEN DREAM

Makes 2 servings

¾ cup water

2 kiwis, peeled
   and quartered

½ cup frozen
   pineapple chunks

½ avocado

1 tablespoon
   chia seeds

Combine water, kiwis, pineapple and avocado in blender; blend until smooth. Add chia seeds; blend until smooth.

# CREAMY CHOCOLATE SMOOTHIE

Makes 1 serving

1 cup unsweetened
   almond milk

1 frozen banana

½ avocado

1 tablespoon
   unsweetened
   cocoa powder

1 tablespoon honey

Combine almond milk, banana, avocado, cocoa and honey in blender; blend until smooth.

Kiwi Green Dream

# RUBY RED DELIGHT

Makes 2 servings

¼ cup water

1 navel orange,
   peeled and seeded

1 medium beet, peeled
   and cut into chunks

½ cup seedless
   red grapes

½ cup frozen
   strawberries

¼ teaspoon
   ground ginger

Combine water, orange, beet, grapes, strawberries and ginger in blender; blend until smooth.

# TANGY APPLE KALE SMOOTHIE

Makes 3 servings

1 cup water

2 Granny Smith apples,
   seeded and cut into
   chunks

2 cups baby kale

1 frozen banana

Combine water, apples, kale and banana in blender; blend until smooth.

Ruby Red Delight

# GREEN PINEAPPLE PICK-ME-UP

## Makes 1 serving

½ cup frozen
    pineapple chunks

½ avocado

1 cup baby kale

1 tablespoon lime juice

1 teaspoon honey

Combine pineapple, avocado, kale, lime juice and honey in blender; blend until smooth.

# BANANA CHAI SMOOTHIE

## Makes 2 servings

¾ cup water

¼ cup unsweetened
    coconut milk
    beverage

2 frozen bananas

1 teaspoon honey

¼ teaspoon
    ground ginger

¼ teaspoon
    ground cinnamon

¼ teaspoon vanilla

    Pinch ground cloves
    (optional)

Combine water, coconut milk, bananas, honey, ginger, cinnamon, vanilla and cloves, if desired, in blender; blend until smooth.

Green Pineapple
Pick-Me-Up

# JUST PEACHY CANTALOUPE SMOOTHIE

Makes 2 servings

¼ cup orange juice

2 cups frozen
   sliced peaches

1½ cups cantaloupe
   chunks

1 tablespoon
   almond butter

Combine orange juice, peaches, cantaloupe and almond butter in blender; blend until smooth.

# BERRY CRANBERRY BLAST

Makes 2 servings

1 cup water

1 cup frozen
   mixed berries

½ cup fresh or thawed
   frozen cranberries

½ avocado

1 tablespoon honey

½ teaspoon grated
   fresh ginger

Combine water, mixed berries, cranberries, avocado, honey and ginger in blender; blend until smooth.

Just Peachy
Cantaloupe
Smoothie

# SUPER C SMOOTHIE
## Makes 3 servings

⅔ cup water

2 navel oranges, peeled and seeded

2 cups frozen blackberries

2 cups baby kale

1 avocado

2 tablespoons honey

Combine water, oranges, blackberries, kale, avocado and honey in blender; blend until smooth.

# SPA SMOOTHIE
## Makes 1 serving

½ cup diced peeled cucumber

½ cup peeled cantaloupe chunks

½ cup sliced fresh strawberries

½ cup ice cubes

Grated peel and juice of 1 lemon

1 tablespoon honey

Combine cucumber, cantaloupe, strawberries, ice, lemon peel, lemon juice and honey in blender; blend until smooth.

Super C Smoothie

# CINNAMON SQUASH PEAR SMOOTHIE

Makes 1 serving

1 pear, seeded and
   cut into chunks
¾ cup frozen cooked
   winter squash
1 teaspoon honey
¼ teaspoon ground
   cinnamon

Combine pear, squash, honey and cinnamon in blender; blend until smooth.

# CHERRY ALMOND SMOOTHIE

Makes 2 servings

½ cup almond milk
1½ cups frozen dark
   sweet cherries
½ banana
2 teaspoons
   almond butter
⅛ teaspoon
   ground cinnamon

Combine almond milk, cherries, banana, almond butter and cinnamon in blender; blend until smooth.

Cinnamon
Squash
Pear
Smoothie

# BLUEBERRY CHERRY BLEND

Makes 2 servings

¾ cup water

¾ cup frozen
   blueberries

¾ cup frozen dark
   sweet cherries

½ avocado

1 tablespoon
   lemon juice

1 teaspoon
   ground flaxseed

Combine water, blueberries, cherries, avocado, lemon juice and flaxseed in blender; blend until smooth.

# GREENS GALORE

Makes 2 servings

¼ cup water

2 small Granny Smith
   apples, seeded and
   cut into chunks

1 cup baby spinach

⅓ seedless cucumber,
   peeled and cut
   into chunks
   (4-inch piece)

¼ cup ice cubes

⅓ cup fresh mint leaves
   (about 3 sprigs)

Combine water, apples, spinach, cucumber, ice and mint in blender; blend until smooth.

Blueberry Cherry Blend

# TROPICAL STORM SMOOTHIE

Makes 2 servings

¼ cup water

1 cup peeled papaya chunks

1 cup frozen pineapple chunks

½ frozen banana

1 tablespoon lemon juice

⅛ teaspoon ground cinnamon

Combine water, papaya, pineapple, banana, lemon juice and cinnamon in blender; blend until smooth.

# PUMPKIN POWER SMOOTHIE

Makes 1 serving

⅓ cup water

1 sweet red apple, seeded and cut into chunks

½ frozen banana

½ cup canned pumpkin

½ cup ice cubes

1 tablespoon lemon juice

1 tablespoon ground flaxseed

1 teaspoon honey

Dash ground nutmeg

Combine water, apple, banana, pumpkin, ice, lemon juice, flaxseed, honey and nutmeg in blender; blend until smooth.

Tropical
Storm
Smoothie

# METRIC CONVERSION CHART

## VOLUME MEASUREMENTS (dry)

1/8 teaspoon = 0.5 mL
1/4 teaspoon = 1 mL
1/2 teaspoon = 2 mL
3/4 teaspoon = 4 mL
1 teaspoon = 5 mL
1 tablespoon = 15 mL
2 tablespoons = 30 mL
1/4 cup = 60 mL
1/3 cup = 75 mL
1/2 cup = 125 mL
2/3 cup = 150 mL
3/4 cup = 175 mL
1 cup = 250 mL
2 cups = 1 pint = 500 mL
3 cups = 750 mL
4 cups = 1 quart = 1 L

## VOLUME MEASUREMENTS (fluid)

1 fluid ounce (2 tablespoons) = 30 mL
4 fluid ounces (1/2 cup) = 125 mL
8 fluid ounces (1 cup) = 250 mL
12 fluid ounces (1 1/2 cups) = 375 mL
16 fluid ounces (2 cups) = 500 mL

## WEIGHTS (mass)

1/2 ounce = 15 g
1 ounce = 30 g
3 ounces = 90 g
4 ounces = 120 g
8 ounces = 225 g
10 ounces = 285 g
12 ounces = 360 g
16 ounces = 1 pound = 450 g

## DIMENSIONS

1/16 inch = 2 mm
1/8 inch = 3 mm
1/4 inch = 6 mm
1/2 inch = 1.5 cm
3/4 inch = 2 cm
1 inch = 2.5 cm

## OVEN TEMPERATURES

250°F = 120°C
275°F = 140°C
300°F = 150°C
325°F = 160°C
350°F = 180°C
375°F = 190°C
400°F = 200°C
425°F = 220°C
450°F = 230°C

## BAKING PAN SIZES

| Utensil | Size in Inches/Quarts | Metric Volume | Size in Centimeters |
|---|---|---|---|
| Baking or Cake Pan (square or rectangular) | 8×8×2 | 2 L | 20×20×5 |
| | 9×9×2 | 2.5 L | 23×23×5 |
| | 12×8×2 | 3 L | 30×20×5 |
| | 13×9×2 | 3.5 L | 33×23×5 |
| Loaf Pan | 8×4×3 | 1.5 L | 20×10×7 |
| | 9×5×3 | 2 L | 23×13×7 |
| Round Layer Cake Pan | 8×1½ | 1.2 L | 20×4 |
| | 9×1½ | 1.5 L | 23×4 |
| Pie Plate | 8×1¼ | 750 mL | 20×3 |
| | 9×1¼ | 1 L | 23×3 |
| Baking Dish or Casserole | 1 quart | 1 L | — |
| | 1½ quart | 1.5 L | — |
| | 2 quart | 2 L | — |